The Sociology and Politics of Health

T0173796

Health care systems, the role of health professionals and the experience of health and illness are all undergoing change and development as we enter the twenty-first century. *The Sociology and Politics of Health* is a collection of key readings through which to explore the sociological and political dimensions of health, illness and health care. Combining classic pieces with more up-to-date contributions it includes examples taken from current domestic and international initiatives and draws on humanist, materialist, feminist and constructionalist perspectives. *The Sociology and Politics of Health* covers:

- ideology and policy
- social stratification
- professionalisation
- the experience of health and illness

This reader offers health studies students, nurses and other health professionals an invaluable introduction to an increasingly important field of social inquiry.

Michael Purdy is Lecturer in Nursing at the University of Sheffield. **David Banks** is Senior Lecturer in the School of Health at the University of Teeside.

The Sociology and Politics of Health

A reader

Edited by
Michael Purdy and
David Banks

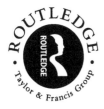

London and New York

First published 2001
by Routledge
11 New Fetter Lane, London EC4P 4EE

Simultaneously published in the USA and Canada
by Routledge
29 West 35th Street, New York, NY 10001

Routledge is an imprint of the Taylor & Francis Group

Publisher's note: ellipses in brackets denote an editorial omission from the original text

Typeset in Galliard by Exe Valley Dataset Ltd

British Library Cataloguing in Publication Data
A catalogue record for this book is available from the British Library

Library of Congress Cataloging in Publication Data
The sociology and politics of health: a reader/edited by Michael Purdy and David Banks.
    p. cm.
    Includes bibliographical references and index.
    1. Social medicine. 2. Medical policy–Social aspects. 3. Medicine–Political aspects. I. Purdy,
Michael, 1953– II. Banks, David, 1956–

RA418 .S6737 2001
362.1′0941-dc21   00-051818

ISBN 0-415-23318-6 (hbk)
ISBN 0-415-23319-4 (pbk)

Contents

PART II
Social stratification and health 59

PART III
Professionalisation and health 123

Acknowledgements

The editors and publishers wish to thank the following for permission to use copyright material:

Allen & Unwin for material from Wendy Seymour's 'Containing the body' from *Health Matters: A Sociology of Illness, Prevention and Care*, ed. A. Petersen and C. Waddell (1998) pp. 156–68; Edward Arnold for material from Thomas McKeown, *The Modern Rise of Population* (1976); Colin Barnes for his article 'Disability and the Myth of the Independent Researcher', *Disability and Society*, 11: 1 (1996) pp. 107–10, and from *Disability Studies: Past, Present and Future*, ed. L. Barton and M. Oliver (1997), The Disability Press, pp. 239–43; Baywood Publishing Company for material from Robert Crawford, 'You are dangerous to your health: the ideology and politics of victim blaming', *International Journal of Health Services*, 7: 4 (1977) pp. 663–80; Blackwell Publishers Ltd and the Editorial Board of *Sociology of Health & Illness* for material from David Armstrong, 'The rise of surveillance medicine', *Sociology of Health & Illness*, 17: 3 (1995) pp. 393–404, Mel Bartley, David Blane and George Davey Smith, 'Introduction: beyond the Black Report', *Sociology of Health & Illness*, 20: 5 (1998) pp. 563–77, and Hazel MacRae, 'Managing courtesy stigma: the case of Alzheimer's disease', *Sociology of Health & Illness*, 21: 1 (1999) pp. 54–70; *British Medical Journal* for permission to reproduce Peter Phillimore, Alastair Beattie and Peter Townsend, 'Widening inequality of health in northern England 1981–91', *British Medical Journal*, 308 (1994) pp. 1125–8; The University of Chicago Press and Eliot Freidson for material from his *Profession of Medicine: A Study of the Sociology of Applied Knowledge* (1970); The Controller of Her Majesty's Stationery Office for permission to reproduce extracts from the following Crown copyright material, Sir Douglas Black (chairman), *Inequalities in Health – Report of a Research Working Group*, 1980, Secretaries of State for Health, *Working for Patients* (Cm. 555) (1989), Secretary of State for Health, *The New NHS – Modern, Dependable* (Cm. 3807) (1997), Sir Donald Acheson (chairman), *Independent Inquiry into Inequalities in Health Report* (1998), Home Office, *Supporting Families – A Consultation Document* (1998), and Secretary of State for Health, *Saving Lives: Our Healthier Nation* (Cm. 4386) (1999); Elsevier Science Ltd for permission to reproduce Irving Kenneth Zola, 'Pathways to the doctor – from person to patient', *Social Science & Medicine*, 7 (1973) pp. 677–89; David Green for material from his *Everyone A Private Patient: An Analysis of the Structural Flaws in the NHS and How They Could be Remedied*, The Institute of Economic Affairs (1988); Macmillan Press Ltd for material from Lesley Doyal, *What Makes Women Sick: Gender and the Political Economy of Health* (1995); Beverley McNamara for her chapter 'A good enough death' from *Health Matters: A Sociology of Illness, Prevention and Care*, ed. A. Petersen and C. Waddell (1998) pp. 169–84, Allen & Unwin/Open University Press; Routledge for material from Mildred Blaxter, *Health and Lifestyles* (1990), Hilary Graham, 'Researching women's health work: a study of the lifestyles of women on income support' from *Working for Equality in Health*, ed. P. Bywaters and E. McLeod (1996) pp. 161–78, F.A. Hayek, *The Road to Serfdom* (1944) (reprinted 1976 by Routledge & Kegan Paul), David J. Hunter, 'From tribalism to corporatism: the managerial challenge to medical dominance' from *Challenging Medicine*, ed. J. Gabe, D. Kellcher and G. Williams (1994) pp. 1–22, and Terry Johnson, 'Governmentalty and the institutionalization of expertise' from *Health Professions and the State in Europe*, ed. T. Johnson, G. Larkin and M. Saks (1995) pp. 7–24; Sage Publications Ltd and Mike Featherstone for material from his 'The body in consumer society', *Theory, Culture & Society*, 1: 2 (1982) pp. 18–33, and Sage Publications Ltd and Deborah Lupton for material from her *The Imperative of Health: Public Health and the Regulated Body* (1995); Gerry Stimson and Barbara Webb for material from their *Going to See the Doctor: The Consultation Process in General Practice*, Routledge & Kegan Paul (1975); Peter Townsend for material from his and Brian Abel-Smith's, *The Poor and the Poorest: A New Analysis of the Ministry of Labour's Family Expenditure Surveys of 1953–54 and 1960*, Bell & Sons Ltd (1965); World Health Organisation for material from *The World Health Report 1999 – Making a Difference*.

Every effort has been made to trace all the copyright-holders, but if any have been inadvertently overlooked the publishers will be pleased to make the necessary arrangement at the first opportunity.

General introduction

The sociology and politics of health is a well-established field of social enquiry. Its significance to anyone wishing to understand the complexities of health, illness and health care practice is likely to increase as we move into the twenty-first century and as health care systems, the role of health professionals and the experience of health and illness continue to be subject to significant change and development. The impact on health care of the radical restructuring of the welfare state, the implications for the role of health professionals of mounting challenges to their authority over health matters, and the effects on personal experience of an imperative of personal responsibility for health and illness are all examples of the scale and scope of change in the health field. With its ability to critically situate health, illness and health care systems in a wider socio-economic and historical context, a sociology and politics of health offers an essential perspective with which to examine the turbulent contemporary health scene in the United Kingdom. This collection of readings is designed to offer health professionals, and in particular nurses, a resource for exploring sociological and political dimensions of health, illness and health care.

Sociology is an essential part of nursing practice since health and social care are always delivered to individual patients and clients in a social context. In working with an individual patient or client the nurse is working with a person whose health care needs are very much affected, if not determined, by the social and cultural processes in which their unique life takes shape, develops and changes. Having a sociological perspective sensitises the nurse to social and political features of health and illness and of the health care systems in which their practice takes place. Such a perspective emphasises that as health care professionals we should be concerned with delivering care to populations and not just to individual patients. In other words, a sociological perspective emphasises the public health role of *all* nurses. It ensures that public health issues and challenges are not ignored and enables the nurse to recognise social inequalities in health and health care and act to reduce them. A sociological perspective confirms that as nurses we need to recognise that our humanitarian commitment to individualised patient care is only achievable if high quality care is provided for everyone (Purdy 1996).

The significance of a sociology and politics of health to the practice of health professionals is increasing as we move into the twenty-first century. Modernisation plans for the National Health Service (Secretary of State for Health 1997, 2000) challenge traditional professional boundaries, call for health services to be more responsive to the needs of users and place equity in health care and the need to reduce inequalities in health at the centre of current policy and health care provision. This radical agenda demands that all health professionals develop a public health perspective in their work, with nurses, health visitors and midwives being recognised as having a crucial contribution to make in addressing the effects of poverty and tackling health inequalities and social exclusion (DOH 1999a, 1999b).

In developing new roles and meeting the changing expectations of both government and users of health services, nurses and other health professionals will find in a sociology and politics of health a *critical* perspective with which to explore issues of health, illness and health care. For a defining characteristic of sociology is its critical capacity. As Peter Berger stated almost forty years ago, 'It can be said that the first wisdom of sociology is this – things are not what they seem' (1963: 34). To be critical is not, however, to be dismissive of the views, accounts and beliefs regarding health and illness which health professionals and users of health services hold. Rather, it is to question the views which common sense simply urges us to accept too easily. The aim of this Reader is to aid that questioning.

The choice of readings combines a selection of 'classic' pieces with contemporary contributions, including examples taken from current domestic and international initiatives in the field of health and social policy. The relevance of the various approaches which social theory has brought to bear on the sociology and politics of health, and for understanding health in the new millennium, is demonstrated by including contributions drawn from humanist, materialist, feminist and constructionalist perspectives. The readings are organised into four distinct but related themes that reflect the significant changes and developments affecting contemporary health care systems, the role of health professionals and the experience of health and illness in the late twentieth century. The four themes are: (i) *ideology and policy* – the impact of significant political and ideological shifts in the late twentieth century has been to call into question state welfarism and a 'collectivist' National Health Service built on principles of social justice; (ii) *social stratification and health* – despite half a century of state welfarism, continued and growing 'inequalities of health' reflect the salience of various dimensions of social stratification on health, illness and access to health care services; (iii) *professionalisation and health* – during the twentieth century, health has become professionalised and medical hegemony established, yet there are increasing challenges to professionalisation and medicalisation which are growing in strength as we enter the twenty-first century; and, (iv) *experiencing health and illness* – against the backdrop of rapid social, cultural and economic change which has characterised Western societies at the close of the century, individuals and populations 'enjoy' increasingly varied experiences of health and illness. Other themes and issues are addressed by specific readings and the relationship and significance of these to the four major themes is highlighted and detailed in the editors' introduction to each section of the Reader.

References

Berger, P.L. (1963 [1991]) *Invitation to Sociology: A Humanistic Perspective*, Harmondsworth: Penguin.
Department of Health (DOH) (1999a) *Reducing Health Inequalities: an Action Report*, London: DOH.
—— (1999b) *Making a Difference: Strengthening the Nursing, Midwifery and Health Visiting Contribution to Health and Healthcare*, London: DOH.
Purdy, M. (1996) 'Is nursing anti-social?', *Nursing Times* 92, 20: 42–4.
Secretary of State for Health (1997) *The New NHS – Modern, Dependable*, Cm. 3807, London: The Stationery Office.
—— (2000) *The NHS Plan – A Plan for Investment, A Plan for Reform*, Cm. 4818-1, London: The Stationery Office.

Part I
Ideology and policy

Introduction

The readings in this section are concerned with the broad ideological and political context in which the National Health Service (NHS) has been founded, developed and is expected to change as we move into the twenty-first century. For excellent commentary on the history and development of the NHS since 1948 see, for example, Klein (1995), Rivett (1998), Webster (1998) and Berridge (1999). Two ideological traditions, 'collectivism' and 'individualism', have been responsible for the development of health policy over the last half-century in the United Kingdom. These are paired here with examples taken from the policy initiatives, which they have each generated.

The basis of 'collectivism' and the programmes of social welfarism which it gave rise to in the twentieth century is to be found in the condemnation of the social effects of rapid industrialisation and urbanisation which signalled the evolution of early industrial capitalism in the nineteenth century. The devastating effects on the health and welfare of the urban masses on which the new economic system depended are graphically illustrated here by an extract (Reading 1) from Engels' critique of the factory system in England. Engels' materialist analysis argues that the poor health and premature deaths of the English working class are caused by their conditions of life, conditions over which they have no control but which are determined by the demands of an economic system based on unrestrained exploitation and competition. It followed that if poor health was socially determined then society could improve health by improving the conditions of life of the population. The horrific conditions which Engels describes clearly provided an impetus for the public health movement of the late nineteenth century, although the extent to which such social (collective) intervention reflected a new-found benevolence on the part of the ruling class and state or served their economic self-interest, by securing a healthier workforce and armed force, is open to debate.

By the middle of the twentieth century, collectivist principles of social justice were being embraced by many Western democracies and the era of state welfarism began. In Britain the end of the Second World War saw cross-party consensus on the need for a 'welfare state', a central component of which was a National Health Service (NHS). The collectivist principles of social justice which informed health and welfare policy during this period are found in the extract reproduced here (Reading 2) from the 1946 NHS Bill which provided a 'summary of the proposed new service'. A 'comprehensive' health service was to be established, available to all regardless of 'financial means, age, sex, employment or vocation, area of residence, or insurance qualification', and free at the point of delivery. Whilst the NHS, which emerged on 5 July 1948, was very much the product of political compromise and accommodation to the self-interest of the medical profession, it nevertheless established a collectivist agenda at the heart of government policymaking. This agenda was to remain virtually intact for thirty years.

Challenges to collectivism have a longer history. Critics of the 'social engineering' which state welfarism was seen to require and of the dehumanising aspects of state bureaucracies associated with socialist and communist regimes countered the collectivist ideals of social justice with those of individual freedom of choice, illustrated here (Reading 3) with an extract taken from Hayek's classic 1944 rejection of socialism and advocacy of individual freedoms. For Hayek, the individualist tradition had created Western civilisation. Since the seventeenth century, the increasing emphasis on the freedom and liberty of the individual from political constraints had permitted the growth of commerce, science and capitalist enterprise. In collectivism, Hayek sees a threat to individual freedom and liberty as the state seeks to direct social forces in the pursuit of an 'equal distribution of wealth' rather than allow the free competition of the market to unfold. Hayek restates the fundamental principle of liberalism, 'that in the ordering of our affairs we should make as much use as possible of the spontaneous forces of society, and resort as little as possible to coercion' (*The Road to Serfdom*, p. 13), and argues that the proper role for the state is to limit its activity to securing through its legislative apparatus the conditions for the market mechanism to operate, and, where competition cannot function, to supplement the provision of services.

Such ideas became politically acceptable in the UK with the election to office of a Tory government under the leadership of Margaret Thatcher in 1979 and the ending of the cross-party consensus on state welfarism which this signalled. Driven by economic imperatives, which challenged the continued viability of state welfarism in the late twentieth century, neo-liberalist ideas gained currency once again with individualism replacing collectivism as the ideological framework structuring health and social policy. The impact of this 'New Right' thinking on health policy led to the increasing marketisation of health care and is represented here by an extract taken from the Conservative government's 1989 White Paper *Working For Patients* (Reading 4), which detailed the setting up of an 'internal market' in the NHS in a bid to secure the '3Es' of efficiency, economy and effectiveness. Whilst radical in its restructuring of the NHS and separation of 'purchaser' and 'provider' functions in order to create the conditions for market competition, the Conservative government remained publicly committed to an NHS available to all regardless of income, and financed from general taxation. This continued commitment to funding the NHS from general taxation following the extensive NHS Review of 1988 is a clear indication of the extent to which the NHS reforms represent a political compromise by the government of its ideological stance. This can be gauged from an example of work from the government's Think Tank at the Institute of Economic Affairs (Reading 5). Here, David Green proposes as a solution to the financial crisis of the NHS, which manifested itself in the ward closures, lengthening waiting lists and staff demoralisation of the 1980s, and precipitated Margaret Thatcher's call for the NHS Review, that the service should be funded not from general taxation but rather from private insurance, with government assistance in the form of vouchers to cover the cost of a minimum package of health care services being provided for the poor. Such an insurance-based system would, according to Green, offer both rich and poor alike more choice in the health care they accessed and received, and lead to a more efficient and cost-effective system as 'priced demand' for health care replaced 'unpriced expectations'.

The restructuring of state welfarism, including health care, has continued following the election of a New Labour government in May 1997. Labour's landslide victory heralded the appearance of a third major ideological force informing thinking and policy on health, health care and the wider social and welfare agendas. 'Communitarianism' represents a rejection of both collectivist and individualist 'world views' and seeks to avoid both the rampant self-serving dogma of the market and the collectivist excesses of 'nanny state' social engineering. The 'communitarian agenda' emphasises the need for individual social responsibility and locates a renewed commitment to social solidarity in the institutions of civil society, and particularly in the 'family' and 'community' (Etzioni 1993). At the policy interface the impact of communitarianism on New Labour's policy agenda is illustrated by an extract (Reading 6) taken from the 1998 Home Office consultative document *Supporting Families*. In this document the government emphasises the role of the family at the heart of society, and whilst recognising 'that families are, and will always be, mainly shaped by private choices well beyond the influence of government' (p. 5), argues that government must nevertheless do what it can to support and strengthen this core social institution at a time when it is under stress. The crisis in the family is seen by the government to be reflected in the rising divorce rate, increasing numbers of single parent households, more child poverty, and rising crime and drug abuse which 'are indirect symptoms of problems in the family'. A range of measures are identified to support and strengthen families – including the development of an 'enhanced role' for health visitors, the funding of *Sure Start* programmes (DfEE 1999) and the setting up of a national parenting help line – and to enable parents to better discharge their responsibilities.

Communitarianism's 'third way' promises to provide the ideological and political 'world view' for health, health care and the experience of health and illness deep into the twenty-first century. Its impact on national and international health policy is represented in this collection by three readings.

Reading 7 from New Labour's 1997 White Paper on the *New NHS* signals the government's intention to rebuild a modern NHS for the twenty-first century which avoids both a return to the 'command and control' culture of the 1970s or a perpetuation of a public health service operating according to free market principles. The White Paper sets out the plans for replacing the 'internal market' with a system of 'integrated care' which is responsive to the needs of patients and 'based on partnership and driven by performance'. New Labour envisages a ten-year programme of 'evolutionary change' which retains certain key elements of the system inherited from the Conservative administration that work, and which installs co-operation rather than competition as the principal mechanism for achieving improvements in both quality of service and cost effectiveness. A primary care-led NHS is the government's goal and the *New NHS* details the structural changes, including the development of 'primary care groups', which it sees as essential to achieving this.

Labour's retention of key elements of the Tory reforms, in particular the purchaser/provider split, demonstrates the inherent pragmatism of the 'third way', keeping those 'New Right' elements which make economic sense whilst dispensing with the ideological basis of the initial welfare consensus. Reading 8 lays out the basis of a new consensus in the context of public health. This extract from the 1999 White Paper on Public Health argues that far from 'blaming the victim' for poor lifestyle choices, government should seek to establish and build a partnership in which individuals, families, communities and government all recognise and act in terms of their social responsibilities and obligations rather than purely in terms of their individual rights. A new consensus may be found in a 'contract for health' involving 'a three-way partnership between people, local communities and government'.

The new emerging consensus of the third way signals a 'new universalism' in the field of health for the twenty-first century. This is represented here (Reading 9) by the World Health Organisation's call in 1999 for governments to increasingly target resources at those groups with the poorest health rather than attempt to provide universal care for all. Rationing is seen to be not only inevitable but also desirable in this 'new universalism', which combines 'universalism with economic realism'. According to the World Health Organisation, 'classic universalism' failed to recognise both 'resource limits and the limits to government' whilst approaches to health based on free market principles ration services according to 'the ability to pay'. In the new century, government will provide leadership and finance the health care system, with services being offered by many different types of provider and 'open and informed debate' deciding health priorities and identifying 'lower priority services' which individuals will need to purchase. In the twenty-first century, universalism is redefined to mean 'coverage for all; not coverage of everything'.

References

Berridge, V. (1999) *Health and Society in Britain Since 1939*, Cambridge: Cambridge University Press.

Department for Education and Employment (DfEE) (1999) *Sure Start: Making a Difference for Children and Families*, London: DfEE.

Etzioni, A. (1993) *The Spirit of Community: Rights, Responsibilities and the Communitarian Agenda*, London: Fontana Press.

Klein, R. (1995) *The New Politics of the NHS*, 3rd edition, London: Longman.

Rivett, G (1998) *From Cradle to Grave: Fifty Years of the NHS*, London: King's Fund.

Webster, C. (1998) *The NHS: A Political History*, Oxford: Oxford University Press.

1 The condition of the working class in England*

Frederick Engels

When one individual inflicts bodily injury upon another, such injury that death results, we call the deed manslaughter; when the assailant knew in advance that the injury would be fatal, we call his deed murder. But when society[1] places hundreds of proletarians in such a position that they inevitably meet a too early and an unnatural death, one which is quite as much a death by violence as that by the sword or bullet; when it deprives thousands of the necessaries of life, places them under conditions in which they *cannot* live – forces them, through the strong arm of the law, to remain in such conditions until that death ensues which is the inevitable consequence – knows that these thousands of victims must perish, and yet permits these conditions to remain, its deed is murder just as surely as the deed of the single individual; disguised, malicious murder, murder against which none can defend himself, which does not seem what it is, because no man sees the murderer, because the death of the victim seems a natural one, since the offence is more one of omission than of commission. But murder it remains. I have now to prove that society in England daily and hourly commits what the working-men's organs, with perfect correctness, characterize as social murder, that it has placed the workers under conditions in which they can neither retain health nor live long; that it undermines the vital force of these workers gradually, little by little, and so hurries them to the grave before their time. I have further to prove that society knows how injurious such conditions are to the health and the life of the workers, and yet does nothing to improve these conditions. That it *knows* the consequences of its deeds; that its act is, therefore, not mere manslaughter, but murder, I shall have proved, when I cite official documents, reports of Parliament and of the Government, in substantiation of my charge.

That a class which lives under the conditions already sketched and is so ill-provided with the most necessary means of subsistence, cannot be healthy and can reach no advanced age, is self-evident. Let us review the circumstances once more with especial reference to the health of the workers. The centralization of population in great cities exercises of itself an unfavourable

*This is an extract from Engels, F. *The Condition of the Working Class in England*, translated by the Institute of Marxism-Leninism, Moscow, Panther Books, 1969, pp. 27–33.

influence; the atmosphere of London can never be so pure, so rich in oxygen, as the air of the country; two and a half million pairs of lungs, two hundred and fifty thousand fires, crowded upon an area three to four miles square, consume an enormous amount of oxygen, which is replaced with difficulty, because the method of building cities in itself impedes ventilation. The carbonic acid gas, engendered by respiration and fire, remains in the streets by reason of its specific gravity, and the chief air current passes over the roofs of the city. The lungs of the inhabitants fail to receive the due supply of oxygen, and the consequence is mental and physical lassitude and low vitality. For this reason, the dwellers in cities are far less exposed to acute, and especially to inflammatory, affections than rural populations, who live in a free, normal atmosphere; but they suffer the more from chronic affections. And if life in large cities is, in itself, injurious to health, how great must be the harmful influence of an abnormal atmosphere in the working-people's quarters, where, as we have seen, everything combines to poison the air. In the country, it may, perhaps, be comparatively innoxious to keep a dung-heap adjoining one's dwelling, because the air has free ingress from all sides; but in the midst of a large town, among closely built lanes and courts that shut out all movement of the atmosphere, the case is different. All putrefying vegetable and animal substances give off gases decidedly injurious to health, and if these gases have no free way of escape, they inevitably poison the atmosphere. The filth and stagnant pools of the working-people's quarters in the great cities have, therefore, the worst effect upon the public health, because they produce precisely those gases which engender disease; so, too, the exalations from contaminated streams. But this is by no means all. The manner in which the great multitude of the poor is treated by society today is revolting. They are drawn into the large cities where they breathe a poorer atmosphere than in the country; they are relegated to districts which, by reason of the method of construction, are worse ventilated than any others; they are deprived of all means of cleanliness, of water itself, since pipes are laid only when paid for, and the rivers so polluted that they are useless for such purposes; they are obliged to throw all offal and garbage, all dirty water, often all disgusting drainage and excrement into the streets, being without other means of disposing of them; they are thus compelled to infect the region of their own dwellings. Nor is this enough. All conceivable evils are heaped upon the heads of the poor. If the population of great cities is too dense in general, it is they in particular who are packed into the least space. As though the vitiated atmosphere of the streets were not enough, they are penned in dozens into single rooms, so that the air they breathe at night is enough in itself to stifle them. They are given damp dwellings, cellar dens that are not waterproof from below, or garrets that leak from above. Their houses are so built that the clammy air cannot escape. They are supplied bad, tattered, or rotten clothing, adulterated and indigestible food. They are exposed to the most exciting changes of mental condition, the most violent vibrations between hope and fear; they are hunted like game, and not permitted to attain peace of mind and quiet enjoyment of life. They are deprived of all enjoyments except that of sexual indulgence and drunkenness, are worked every day to the point of complete exhaustion of their mental and physical energies, and are thus constantly spurred on to the maddest excess in the only two enjoyments at their command. And if they surmount all this, they fall victims to want of work in a crisis when all the little is taken from them that had hitherto been vouchsafed them.

How is it possible, under such conditions, for the lower class to be healthy and long lived? What else can be expected than an excessive mortality, an unbroken series of epidemics, a progressive deterioration in the physique of the working population? Let us see how the facts stand.

That the dwellings of the workers in the worst portions of the cities, together with the other conditions of life of this class, engender numerous diseases, is attested on all sides. The article already quoted from the *Artisan* asserts with perfect truth, that lung diseases must be the inevitable consequence of such conditions, and that, indeed, cases of this kind are disproportionately frequent in this class. That the bad air of London, and especially of the working-people's districts, is in the highest degree favourable to the development of consumption, the hectic appearance of great numbers of persons sufficiently indicates. If one roams the streets a little in the early morning, when the multitudes are on their way to their work, one is amazed at the number of persons who look wholly or half-consumptive. Even in Manchester the people have not the same appearance; these pale, lank, narrow-chested, hollow-eyed ghosts, whom one passes at every step, these languid, flabby faces, incapable of the slightest energetic expression, I have seen in such startling numbers only in London, though consumption carries off a horde of victims annually in the factory towns of the North. In competition with consumption stands typhus, to say nothing of scarlet fever, a disease which brings most frightful devastation into the ranks of the working-class. Typhus, that universally diffused affliction, is attributed by the official report on the sanitary condition of the working-class, directly to the bad state of the dwellings in the matters of ventilation, drainage, and cleanliness. This report, compiled, it must not be forgotten, by the leading physicians of England from the testimony of other physicians, asserts that a single ill-ventilated court, a single blind alley without drainage, is enough to engender fever, and usually does engender it, especially if the inhabitants are greatly crowded. This fever has the same character almost everywhere, and develops in nearly every case into specific typhus. It is to be found in the working-people's quarters of all great towns and cities, and in single ill-built, ill-kept streets of smaller places, though it naturally seeks out single victims in better districts also. In London it has now prevailed for a considerable time; its extraordinary violence in the year 1837 gave rise to the report already referred to. According to the annual report of Dr. Southwood Smith on the London Fever Hospital, the number of patients in 1843 was 1,462, or 418 more than in any previous year. In the damp, dirty regions of the north, south, and east districts of London, this disease raged with extraordinary violence. Many of the patients were working-people from the country, who had endured the severest privation while migrating, and, after their arrival, had slept hungry and half-naked in the streets, and so fallen victims to the fever. These people were brought into the hospital in such a state of weakness, that unusual quantities of wine, cognac, and preparations of ammonia and other stimulants were required for their treatment; 16½ per cent of all patients died. This malignant fever is to be found in Manchester; in the worst quarters of the Old Town, Ancoats, Little Ireland, etc., it is rarely extinct; though here, as in the *English* towns generally, it prevails to a less extent than might be expected. In Scotland and Ireland, on the other hand, it rages with a violence that surpasses all conception. In Edinburgh and Glasgow it broke out in 1817, after the famine, and in 1826 and 1837 with especial violence, after the commercial crisis, subsiding somewhat each time after having raged about three years. In Edinburgh about 6,000 persons were attacked by the fever during the epidemic of 1817, and about 10,000 in that of 1837, and not only the number of persons attacked but the violence of the disease increased with each repetition.[2]

But the fury of the epidemic in all former periods seems to have been child's play in comparison with its ravages after the crisis of 1842. One-sixth of the whole indigent population of Scotland was seized by the fever, and the infection was carried by wandering beggars with fearful rapidity from one locality to another. It did not reach the middle and upper classes of the population, yet in two months there were more fever cases than in twelve years before. In Glasgow, twelve per cent of the population were seized in the year 1843; 32,000 persons, of whom thirty-two per cent perished, while this mortality in Manchester and Liverpool does not ordinarily exceed eight per cent. The illness reached a crisis on the seventh and fifteenth days; on the latter, the patient usually became yellow, which our authority[3] regards as an indication that the cause of the malady was to be sought in mental excitement and anxiety. In Ireland, too, these fever epidemics have become domesticated. During twenty-one months of the years 1817–18, 39,000 fever patients passed through the Dublin hospital; and in a more recent year, according to Sheriff Alison,[4] 60,000. In Cork the fever hospital received one-seventh of the population in 1817–18, in Limerick in the same time one-fourth, and in the bad quarter of Waterford, nineteen-twentieths of the whole population were ill of the fever at one time.[5]

When one remembers under what conditions the working-people live, when one thinks how crowded their dwellings are, how every nook and corner swarms with human beings, how sick and well sleep in the same room, in the same bed, the only wonder is that a contagious disease like this fever does not spread yet farther. And when one reflects how little medical assistance the sick have at command, how many are without any medical advice whatsoever, and ignorant of the most ordinary precautionary measures, the mortality seems actually small. Dr. Alison, who has made a careful study of this disease, attributes it directly to the want and the wretched condition of the poor, as in the report already quoted. He asserts that privations and the insufficient satisfaction of vital needs are what prepare the frame for contagion and make the epidemic wide-spread and terrible. He proves that a period of privation, a commercial crisis, or a bad harvest, has each time produced the typhus epidemic in Ireland as in Scotland, and that the fury of the plague has fallen almost exclusively on the working-class. It is a noteworthy fact, that according to his testimony, the majority of persons who perish by typhus are fathers of families, precisely the persons who can least be spared by those dependent upon them; and several Irish physicians whom he quotes bear the same testimony.

Another category of diseases arises directly from the food rather than the dwellings of the workers. The food of the labourer, indigestible enough in itself, is utterly unfit for young children, and he has neither means nor time to get his children more suitable food. Moreover, the custom of giving children spirits, and even opium, is very general; and these two influences, with the rest of the conditions of life prejudicial to bodily development, give rise to the most diverse affections of the digestive organs, leaving lifelong traces behind them. Nearly all workers have stomachs more or less weak, and are yet forced to adhere to the diet which is the root of the evil. How should they know what is to blame for it? And if they knew, how could they obtain a more suitable regimen so long as they cannot adopt a different way of living and are not better educated? But new disease arises during childhood from impaired digestion. Scrofula is almost universal among the working-class, and scrofulous parents have scrofulous children, especially when the original influences continue in full force to operate upon the inherited tendency of the children. A second consequence of this insufficient bodily nourishment, during the years of growth and development, is rachitis, which is extremely common among the children of the working-class. The hardening of the bones is delayed, the development of the skeleton in general is restricted, and deformities of the legs and spinal column are frequent, in addition to the usual rachitic affections. How greatly all these evils are increased by the changes to which the workers are subject in consequence of fluctuations in trade, want of work, and the scanty wages in time of crisis, it is not necessary to dwell upon. Temporary want of sufficient food, to which almost every working-man is exposed at least once in the course of his life, only contributes to intensify the effect of his usually sufficient but bad diet. Children who are half-starved, just when they most need ample and nutritious food – and how many such there are during every crisis and even when trade is at its best – must inevitably become weak, scrofulous and rachitic in a high degree. And that they do become so, their appearance amply shows. The neglect to which the great mass of working-men's children are condemned leaves ineradicable traces and brings the enfeeblement of the whole race of workers with it. Add to this the unsuitable clothing of this class, the impossibility of precautions against colds, the necessity of toiling so long as health permits, want made more dire when sickness appears, and the only too common lack of all medical assistance; and we have a rough idea of the sanitary condition of the English working-class.

Notes

1 When as here and elsewhere I speak of society as a responsible whole, having rights and duties, I mean, of course, the ruling power of society, the class which at present holds social and political control, and bears, therefore, the responsibility for the condition of those to whom it grants no share in such control. This ruling class in England, as in all other civilized countries, is the bourgeoisie. But that this society, and especially the bourgeoisie, is charged with the duty of protecting every member of society, at least, in his life, to see to it, for example, that no one starves, I need not now prove to my *German* readers. If I were writing for the English bourgeoisie, the case would be different. (And so it is now in Germany. Our German capitalists are fully up to the English level, in this respect at least, in the year of grace, 1886.)
2 Dr. Alison. 'Management of the Poor in Scotland.'
3 Alison. 'Principles of Population,' vol. ii.
4 Dr. Alison in an article read before the British Association for the Advancement of Science. October 1844, in York.
5 Dr. Alison, Management of the Poor in Scotland. (*Note in the German edition.*)

2   National Health Service bill*

Ministry of Health

Introductory

1   The Bill provides for the establishment of a comprehensive health service in England and Wales. A further Bill to provide for Scotland will be introduced later.

2   The Bill does not deal in detail with everything involved in the service. It deals with the main structure. Within that structure, further provision will be made by statutory regulations – on lines which the Bill lays down and subject always to the control of Parliament.

Scope of the service

3   The Bill provides for the following kinds of health services: –

(i)   Hospital and specialist services – i.e. all forms of general and special hospital provision, including mental hospitals, together with sanatoria, maternity accommodation, treatment during convalescence, medical rehabilitation and other institutional treatment. These cover in-patient and out-patient services, the latter including clinics and dispensaries operated as part of any specialist service. The advice and services of specialists of all kinds are also to be made available, where necessary, at Health Centres and in the patient's home.

(ii) Health Centres and general practitioner services – i.e. general personal health care by doctors and dentists whom the patient chooses. These personal practitioner services are to be available both from new publicly equipped Health Centres and also from the practitioners' own surgeries.

(iii) Various supplementary services – including midwifery, maternity and child welfare, health visiting, home-nursing, a priority dental service for children and expectant and nursing mothers, domestic help where needed on health grounds, vaccination and immunisation against

---

*This is an abridged extract from Ministry of Health (1946) *National Health Service bill – summary of the proposed new service*, Cmd. 6761, HMSO, pp. 3–5, 9, 14–16.

infectious diseases, additional special care and after-care in cases of illness, ambulance services, blood transfusion and laboratory services. (Special school health services are already provided for in the Education Act of 1944.)

(iv) The provision of spectacles, dentures and other appliances, together with drugs and medicines – at hospitals, Health Centres, clinics, pharmacists' shops and elsewhere, as may be appropriate.

Availability of the service

4　All the services or any part of it, is to be available to everyone in England and Wales. The Bill imposes no limitations on availability – e.g. limitations based on financial means, age, sex, employment or vocation, area of residence, or insurance qualification.

5　The last is important. If the National Insurance Bill now before Parliament is passed into law, almost everyone will become compulsorily insurable, and after payment of the appropriate contributions will become entitled to the various cash benefits – including sickness and maternity benefits – for which that Bill provides. A proportion of their contributions will be used to help to finance the health services under the present Bill, but the various health service benefits under the present Bill are not made conditional upon any insurance qualification or the proof of having paid contributions. There are no waiting or qualifying periods.

6　The service is to be available from a date to be declared by Order in Council under the Bill, and it is hoped that this will be at the beginning of the year 1948.

The service to be free of fees or charges

7　The health service is to be financed partly from the exchequer, partly from local rates, partly from the help (mentioned above) which part of the National Insurance contributions will give. There are to be no fees or charges to the patient, with the following exceptions:–

(i)　There will be some charges (to be prescribed later by regulations) for the renewal or repair of spectacles, dentures and other appliances, where this is made necessary through negligence in the care of the articles provided.

(ii)　There will be charges (taking into account ability to pay) for the provision of domestic help under the Bill and for certain goods or articles (e.g. supplementary foods, blankets, etc.) which may be provided in connection with maternity and child welfare or the special care or after-care of the sick.

(iii) It will be open to people if they wish, in certain cases, to pay for additional amenities within the arrangements of the service – e.g. to pay extra for articles or appliances of higher cost than those normally made available, or to pay charges for private rooms in hospitals (which they will nevertheless be able to obtain free where privacy is medically necessary).

General organisation of the service

8   The Bill places a general duty upon the Minister of Health to promote a comprehensive health service for the improvement of the physical and mental health of the people of England and Wales, and for the prevention, diagnosis and treatment of illness. To bring physical and mental health closer together in a single service, it transfers to the Minister the present administrative functions of the Board of Control in regard to mental health (the Board retaining only its quasi-judicial functions connected with the liberty of the subject).

9   The Bill proposes that the Minister shall discharge his general responsibility through three main channels:–

(a) For parts of the service to be organised on a new national or regional basis – i.e. hospital and specialist services, blood transfusion and bacteriological laboratories for the control of epidemics – the Minister is to assume direct responsibility; but he is to entrust the actual administration of the hospital and specialist services to new regional and local bodies established under the Bill. These bodies are to act on his behalf in suitable areas to be prescribed by him, and they are to include people of practical experience and local knowledge and some with professional qualifications. Special provision is made for hospitals which are the centres of medical and dental teaching.

(b) For parts of the service to be organised as a function of local government – i.e. the provision of new Health Centre premises and a variety of local domiciliary and clinic services – direct responsibility is put upon the major local authorities, the county and county borough councils. They will stand in their ordinary constitutional relationship with the central Ministry, but their general arrangements for these local services are made subject to the Minister's approval.

(c) For the personal practitioner services both in the Health Centres and outside – i.e. the family doctor and dentist and the pharmacist – new local executive machinery is created, in the form of local Executive Councils. One half of the members of each of these Councils will consist of people nominated by the major local authorities and by the Minister, and the other half of people nominated by the local professional practitioners concerned. There will normally be an Executive Council for each of the major local authorities' areas, and they will work within national regulations made by the Minister.

10   By the Minister's side, to provide him with professional and technical guidance, there is to be set up a Central Health Services Council. This

will include people chosen from all the main fields of experience within the service – with various standing committees of experts on particular subjects, medical, dental, nursing and others.

11 Each of these branches of the new organisation is described in more detail in the rest of this paper.

Hospital and specialist service

12 This part of the service covers hospital and consultant services of all kinds, including general and special hospitals, maternity accommodation, tuberculosis sanatoria, infectious diseases units, provision for the chronic sick, mental hospitals and mental deficiency institutions, accommodation for convalescent treatment and medical rehabilitation, and all forms of specialised treatment – e.g. orthopædics, cancer, neuro-surgery, plastic surgery, pædiatrics, gynæcology, ophthalmic services, ear, nose and throat treatment, and others.

[. . .]

General practitioner services

40 This part of the service covers the personal health services provided by general medical practitioners and dentists and the supply of drugs, medicines and appliances.

41 To arrange these services locally new bodies – to be called Executive Councils – are to be established in the area of each county and county borough. As already explained, each Council is to be so composed that one half of its members are professional – appointed by the local doctors, dentists and chemists through their own representative committees in the area – while the other half of the members are to be appointed partly by the local county or county borough council (one third of the Executive Council) and partly by the Minister (one sixth). The Chairman will be appointed by the Minister. Single Executive Councils may sometimes be established for the areas of two or more local authorities.

Health Centres

42 A main feature of the personal practitioner services is to be the development of Health Centres. The object is that the Health Centre system, based on premises technically equipped and staffed at public cost, shall afford facilities both for the general medical and dental services (described immediately below) and also for many of the special clinic services of the local health authorities (described later), and sometimes also for out-post clinics of the hospital and specialist services (already described). Beside forming a base for these services – e.g. providing doctors with equipped and staffed consulting rooms in which to see their

patients – the Centres will also be able to serve as bases for various activities in health education.

43 The Bill makes it the duty of the county and county borough councils to provide, equip, staff and maintain the new Health Centres to the satisfaction of the Minister. The local authorities will directly administer such of their own local clinic facilities as they may provide in the Centres. [. . .]

Local government services

73 This part of the health service comprises the local and domiciliary services which are appropriate to local government, rather than to central government or to any specially devised machinery. The Bill unifies these services in the existing major local authorities – the county and county borough councils – and provides for the formation of joint boards wherever, exceptionally, this may be found desirable.

74 For most of these services, the Bill requires the local health authorities (as they are to be called) to indicate to the Minister the way in which they intend to carry out their responsibilities, and it requires the Minister's general approval. Their proposals, so indicated, are to be made known also to the Regional Boards and Boards of Governors for the hospital service, to the Executive Councils for the general practitioner services, and to any voluntary organisation which to the local authority's knowledge is working in the same field in their area.

75 The purpose of this last requirement is to ensure that these local arrangements are fitted appropriately to the hospital and specialist services for which the Minister is more directly responsible and to the general practitioner services which will be operated within his general regulations and control. This inter-relation between the different arms of the health service is reinforced by the provision (already mentioned) for the local health authorities to nominate one-third of the members of the Executive Councils for the general practitioner services and to be consulted by the Minister in the appointment of Regional Boards, Management Committees and Boards of Governors in the hospital and specialist services. [. . .]

77 The various functions comprised in the local government part of the health service are summarised below.

Maternity and child welfare and midwifery

78 The Bill makes it the duty of every local health authority to make arrangements for the care of expectant and nursing mothers and of children under five years of age who are not attending school and who are there-

fore not covered by the school health service. Their arrangements will include ante-natal clinics for the care of expectant mothers, post-natal and child clinics, the provision of such things as cod-liver oil, fruit juices and other dietary supplements and, in particular, a priority dental service for expectant and nursing mothers and young children.

[. . .]

Health visiting and home nursing

82 It is made the duty of the local health authority to provide for a full health visitor service for all in their area who are sick, or expectant mothers, or those with the care of young children. This widens the present conception of health visiting (as concerned with mothers and children) into a more general service of advice to households where there is sickness or where help of a preventive character may be needed.

83 It is also made the duty of the local health authority to provide a home nursing service for those who – for good reason – need nursing in their own homes.

84 In both of these activities the local authority can, if it likes and if the Minister approves, make all or part of its provision by arrangement with voluntary organisations to act on its behalf.

Local mental health services

85 The main mental treatment and mental deficiency services are to be part of the new hospital and specialist arrangements under the Bill. Local health authorities, however, are given responsibility for all the ordinary local community care in the mental health service – that is to say, the ascertainment of mental defectives and their supervision when they are living in the community. This part of the service covers also the initial proceedings for placing under care those who require treatment under the Lunacy and Mental Treatment Acts.

Vaccination and immunisation

86 Compulsory vaccination is to be abolished by the Bill, but it is to be the duty of the local health authority to provide free vaccination and diphtheria immunisation for anyone who desires them. This service the authority will provide by making arrangements with doctors who are taking part in the general practitioner service – paying appropriate fees to those who undertake it. The vaccines, sera or other preparations required may be supplied without charge by the Minister to local health authorities and doctors and the service may, if circumstances demand, be extended to cover vaccination and immunisation against other diseases beside smallpox and diphtheria.

Ambulance service

87   Apart from vehicles which may need to be provided as part of the hospital service, the provision of the main ambulances and hospital transport required for the health service becomes the duty of the local health authorities, either directly or by arrangement with voluntary organisations. In future the local health authority's ambulances may – and must, if necessary – operate outside their own area.

Care and after-care of the sick

88   Local health authorities are given a new power, and duty where the Minister so requires, to make approved arrangements for the purpose of the prevention of illness and the care and after-care of the sick. This can include such things as the provision of special foods, blankets, extra comforts and special accommodation for invalids and convalescents and the making of grants to voluntary organisations doing work of this kind (but it expressly does not include cash allowances to individuals or families, which is the function of National Insurance). A charge may be made in appropriate cases.

Domestic help

89   Under the existing law local authorities are empowered to provide home helps as part of their maternity and child welfare functions and, during the war, this power has been extended by temporary enactments to enable them to provide domestic help in a wider range of circumstances. The Bill makes this power permanent and extends it to cover the provision of domestic help, subject to the Minister's approval, to any household in which it is needed on grounds of ill-health, maternity, age or the welfare of children. The local health authority will be allowed to make appropriate charge for this service.

3   The road to serfdom*

F. A. Hayek

Individualism and collectivism

> The socialists believe in two things which are absolutely different and
> perhaps even contradictory: freedom and organisation.
>
> Elie Halévy

Before we can progress with our main problem, an obstacle has yet to be
surmounted. A confusion largely responsible for the way in which we are
drifting into things which nobody wants must be cleared up.

This confusion concerns nothing less than the concept of socialism itself. It
may mean, and is often used to describe, merely the ideals of social justice,
greater equality and security which are the ultimate aims of socialism. But it
means also the particular method by which most socialists hope to attain these
ends and which many competent people regard as the only methods by which
they can be fully and quickly attained. In this sense socialism means the
abolition of private enterprise, of private ownership of the means of
production, and the creation of a system of "planned economy" in which the
entrepreneur working for profit is replaced by a central planning body.

There are many people who call themselves socialists although they care
only about the first, who fervently believe in those ultimate aims of socialism
but neither care nor understand how they can be achieved, and who are
merely certain that they must be achieved, whatever the cost. But to nearly all
those to whom socialism is not merely a hope but an object of practical
politics, the characteristic methods of modern socialism are as essential as the
ends themselves. Many people, on the other hand, who value the ultimate
ends of socialism no less than the socialists, refuse to support socialism
because of the dangers to other values they see in the methods proposed by
the socialists. The dispute about socialism has thus become largely a dispute
about means and not about ends – although the question whether the
different ends of socialism can be simultaneously achieved is also involved.

---

*This is an extract from Hayek, F.A. (1944) *The Road to Serfdom*, reprinted 1976 by
Routledge & Kegan Paul, pp. 24–9.

This would be enough to create confusion. And the confusion has been further increased by the common practice of denying that those who repudiate the means value the ends. But this is not all. The situation is still more complicated by the fact that the same means, the "economic planning" which is the prime instrument of socialist reform, can be used for many other purposes. We must centrally direct economic activity if we want to make the distribution of income conform to current ideas of social justice. "Planning", therefore, is wanted by all those who demand that "production for use" be substituted for production for profit. But such planning is no less indispensable if the distribution of incomes is to be regulated in a way which to us appears to be the opposite of just. Whether we should wish that more of the good things of this world should go to some racial élite, the Nordic men, or the members of a party or an aristocracy, the methods which we shall have to employ are the same as those which could ensure an equalitarian distribution.

It may, perhaps, seem unfair to use the term socialism to describe its methods rather than its aims, to use for a particular method a term which for many people stands for an ultimate ideal. It is probably preferable to describe the methods which can be used for a great variety of ends as collectivism and to regard socialism as a species of that genus. Yet, although to most socialists only one species of collectivism will represent true socialism, it must always be remembered that socialism is a species of collectivism and that therefore everything which is true of collectivism as such must apply also to socialism. Nearly all the points which are disputed between socialists and liberals concern the methods common to all forms of collectivism and not the particular ends for which socialists want to use them; and all the consequences with which we shall be concerned in this book follow from the methods of collectivism irrespective of the ends for which they are used. It must also not be forgotten that socialism is not only by far the most important species of collectivism or "planning"; but that it is socialism which has persuaded liberal-minded people to submit once more to that regimentation of economic life which they had overthrown because, in the words of Adam Smith, it puts governments in a position where "to support themselves they are obliged to be oppressive and tyrannical".[1]

*   *   *   *   *

The difficulties caused by the ambiguities of the common political terms are not yet over if we agree to use the term collectivism so as to include all types of "planned economy", whatever the end of planning. The meaning of this term becomes somewhat more definite if we make it clear that we mean that sort of planning which is necessary to realise any given distributive ideals. But as the idea of central economic planning owes its appeal largely to this very vagueness of its meaning, it is essential that we should agree on its precise sense before we discuss its consequences.

"Planning" owes its popularity largely to the fact that everybody desires, of course, that we should handle our common problems as rationally as possible, and that in so doing we should use as much foresight as we can command. In this sense everybody who is not a complete fatalist is a planner, every political act is (or ought to be) an act of planning, and there can be differences only between good and bad, between wise and foresighted and foolish and short-sighted planning. An economist, whose whole task is the study of how men actually do and how they might plan their affairs, is the last person who could object to planning in this general sense. But it is not in this sense that our enthusiasts for a planned society now employ this term, nor merely in this sense that we must plan if we want the distribution of income or wealth to conform to some particular standard. According to the modern planners, and for their purposes, it is not sufficient to design the most rational permanent framework within which the various activities would be conducted by different persons according to their individual plans. This liberal plan, according to them, is no plan – and it is indeed not a plan designed to satisfy particular views about who should have what. What our planners demand is a central direction of all economic activity according to a single plan, laying down how the resources of society should be "consciously directed" to serve particular ends in a definite way.

The dispute between the modern planners and their opponents is, therefore, *not* a dispute on whether we ought to choose intelligently between the various possible organisations of society; it is not a dispute on whether we ought to employ foresight and systematic thinking in planning our common affairs. It is a dispute about what is the best way of so doing. The question is whether for this purpose it is better that the holder of coercive power should confine himself in general to creating conditions under which the knowledge and initiative of individuals is given the best scope so that *they* can plan most successfully; or whether a rational utilisation of our resources requires *central* direction and organisation of all our activities according to some consciously constructed "blueprint". The socialists of all parties have appropriated the term planning for planning of the latter type and it is now generally accepted in this sense. But though this is meant to suggest that this is the only rational way of handling our affairs, it does not of course prove this. It remains the point on which the planners and the liberals disagree.

*   *   *   *   *

It is important not to confuse opposition against this kind of planning with a dogmatic *laissez-faire* attitude. The liberal argument is in favour of making the best possible use of the forces of competition as a means of co-ordinating human efforts, not an argument for leaving things just as they are. It is based on the conviction that where effective competition can be created, it is a better way of guiding individual efforts than any other. It does not deny, but even emphasises, that, in order that competition should work beneficially, a carefully thought-out legal framework is required, and that neither the existing nor the past legal rules are free from grave defects. Nor does it deny that where it is impossible to create the conditions necessary to make competition effective, we must resort to other methods of guiding economic activity. Economic liberalism is opposed, however, to competition being supplanted by inferior methods of co-ordinating individual efforts. And it regards competition as superior not only because it is in most circumstances the most efficient method known, but even more because it is the only method by which our activities can be adjusted to each other without coercive or arbitrary intervention of authority. Indeed, one of the main arguments in favour of competition is that it dispenses with the need for "conscious social control" and that it gives the individuals a chance to decide whether the prospects of a particular occupation are sufficient to compensate for the disadvantages and risks connected with it.

The successful use of competition as the principle of social organisation precludes certain types of coercive interference with economic life, but it admits of others which sometimes may very considerably assist its work and even requires certain kinds of government action. But there is good reason why the negative requirements, the points where coercion must not be used, have been particularly stressed. It is necessary in the first instance that the parties in the market should be free to sell and buy at any price at which they can find a partner to the transaction, and that anybody should be free to produce, sell, and buy anything that may be produced or sold at all. And it is essential that the entry into the different trades should be open to all on equal terms, and that the law should not tolerate any attempts by individuals or groups to restrict this entry by open or concealed force. Any attempt to control prices or quantities of particular commodities deprives competition of its power of bringing about an effective co-ordination of individual efforts, because price changes then cease to register all the relevant changes in circumstances and no longer provide a reliable guide for the individual's actions.

This is not necessarily true, however, of measures merely restricting the allowed methods of production, so long as these restrictions affect all potential producers equally and are not used as an indirect way of controlling prices and quantities. Though all such controls of the methods or production impose extra costs, i.e. make it necessary to use more resources to produce a given output, they may be well worth while. To prohibit the use of certain poisonous substances, or to require special precautions in their use, to limit working hours or to require certain sanitary arrangements, is fully compatible with the preservation of competition. The only question here is whether in the particular instance the advantages gained are greater than the social costs which they impose. Nor is the preservation of competition incompatible with an extensive system of social services – so long as the organisation of these services is not designed in such a way as to make competition ineffective over wide fields.

It is regrettable, though not difficult to explain, that much less attention than to these negative points has in the past been given to the positive require- ments of a successful working of the competitive system. The functioning of competition not only requires adequate organisation of certain institutions like money, markets, and channels of information – some of which can never be adequately provided by private enterprise – but it depends above all on the existence of an appropriate legal system, a legal system designed both to preserve competition and to make it operate as beneficially as possible. It is by no means sufficient that the law should recognise the principle of private property and freedom of contract; much depends on the precise definition of the right of property as applied to different things. The systematic study of the forms of legal institutions which will make the competitive system work efficiently has been sadly neglected; and strong arguments can be advanced that serious shortcomings here, particularly with regard to the law of corporations and of patents, have not only made competition work much more badly than it might have done, but have even led to the destruction of competition in many spheres.

There are, finally, undoubted fields where no legal arrangements can create the main condition on which the usefulness of the system of competition and private property depends: namely, that the owner benefits from all the useful services rendered by his property and suffers for all the damages caused to others by its use. Where, for example, it is impracticable to make the enjoyment of certain services dependent on the payment of a price, competition will not produce the services; and the price system becomes similarly ineffective when the damage caused to others by certain uses of property cannot be effectively charged to the owner of that property. In all these instances there is a divergence between the items which enter into private calculation and those which affect social welfare; and whenever this divergence becomes important some method other than competition may have to be found to supply the services in question. Thus neither the provision of signposts on the roads, nor, in most circumstances, that of the roads themselves, can be paid for by every individual user. Nor can certain harmful effects of deforestation, or of some methods of farming, or of the smoke and noise of factories, be confined to the owner of the property in question or to those who are willing to submit to the damage for an agreed compensation. In such instances we must find some substitute for the regulation by the price mechanism. But the fact that we have to resort to the substitution of direct regulation by authority where the conditions for the proper working of competition cannot be created, does not prove that we should suppress competition where it can be made to function.

To create conditions in which competition will be as effective as possible, to supplement it where it cannot be made effective, to provide the services which, in the words of Adam Smith, "though they may be in the highest degree advantageous to a great society, are, however, of such a nature, that the profit could never repay the expense to any individual or small number of individuals", these tasks provide indeed a wide and unquestioned field for state activity. In no system that could be rationally defended would the state just do nothing. An effective competitive system needs an intelligently designed and continuously adjusted legal framework as much as any other. Even the most essential prerequisite of its proper functioning, the prevention of fraud and deception (including exploitation of ignorance) provides a great and by no means yet fully accomplished object of legislative activity.

Note

1 Quoted in Dugald Stewart's *Memoir of Adam Smith* from a memorandum written by Smith in 1755.

4 Working for patients*

Secretaries of State for Health

Introduction

The achievements of the NHS

1.1 The United Kingdom enjoys high standards of health care. The Health Service has contributed to longer life expectancy, fewer stillbirths and lower rates of perinatal and infant mortality. There have been dramatic increases in the number of people treated in hospital. Transplant surgery is now commonplace. Doctors can carry out successful hip operations on people in their seventies and eighties. People are not only living longer but are enjoying a better quality of life.

1.2 The proposals in this white Paper aim to build on these achievements by providing an even better service for patients. To do that the Government will keep all that is best in the NHS. The principles which have guided it for the last 40 years will continue to guide it into the twenty-first century. The NHS is, and will continue to be, open to all, regardless of income, and financed mainly out of general taxation.

1.3 The NHS is growing at a truly remarkable pace. The number of hospital doctors and dentists has increased from 42,000 in 1978 to over 48,000 in 1987, and the number of nursing and midwifery staff from 444,000 to 514,000. Total gross expenditure will increase from £8 billion in 1978–79 to £26 billion in 1989–90, an increase of 40 per cent after allowing for general inflation. Expenditure by the NHS will then be equivalent to around £35 a week for an average family of four, as compared with about £11 in 1978–79. This and improved productivity mean, to take just one example, that NHS hospital staff now treat over one and a half million more in-patients a year than in 1978, bringing the total to nearly eight million.

The need for change

1.4 Throughout the 1980s the Government has thus presided over a massive expansion of the NHS. It has ensured that the quality of care provided

*This is an abridged extract from Secretaries of State for Health (1989) *Working for Patients*, Cm. 555, The Stationery Office, pp. 2–6, 8–9.

and the response to emergencies remain among the best in the world. But it has become increasingly clear that more needs to be done because of rising demand and an ever-widening range of treatments made possible by advances in medical technology. It has also increasingly been recognised that simply injecting more and more money is not, by itself, the answer.

1.5 It is clear that the organisation of the NHS – the way it delivers health care to the individual patient – also needs to be reformed. The Government has been tackling these organisational problems, and has taken a series of measures to improve the way the NHS is managed. The main one was the introduction of general management from 1984. This is now showing results and has pointed the way ahead.

1.6 New management information systems have provided clear evidence of a wide variation in performance up and down the country. In 1986–87, the average cost of treating acute hospital in-patients varied by as much as 50 per cent between different health authorities, even after allowing for the complexity and mix of cases treated. Similarly, a patient who waits several years for an operation in one place may get that same operation within a few weeks in another. There are wide variations in the drug prescribing habits of GPs, and in some places drug costs are nearly twice as high per head of population as in others. And, at the extremes, there is a twenty-fold variation in the rate at which GPs refer patients to hospital.

1.7 The Government wants to raise the performance of all hospitals and GP practices to that of the best. The main question it has addressed in its review of the NHS has been how best to achieve that. It is convinced that it can be done only by delegating responsibility as closely as possible to where health care is delivered to the patient – predominantly to the GP and the local hospital. Experience in both the public service and the private sector has shown that the best run services are those in which local staff are given responsibility for responding to local needs.

1.8 This White Paper presents a programme of action, summarised in chapter 13, to secure two objectives:

- to give patients, wherever they live in the UK, better health care and greater choice of the services available; and
- greater satisfaction and rewards for those working in the NHS who successfully respond to local needs and preferences.

The Government's proposals

Key changes

1.9 The Government is proposing seven key measures to achieve these objectives:
First: **to make the Health Service more responsive to the needs of patients, as much power and responsibility as possible will be delegated to local level.** This includes the delegation of functions from

Regions to Districts, and from Districts to hospitals. The detailed proposals are set out in the next chapter. They include greater flexibility in setting the pay and conditions of staff, and financial incentives to make the best use of a hospital's assets.

Second: **to stimulate a better service to the patient, hospitals will be able to apply for a new self-governing status as NHS Hospital Trusts.** This means that, while remaining within the NHS, they will take fuller responsibility for their own affairs, harnessing the skills and dedication of their staff. NHS Hospital Trusts will earn revenue from the services they provide. They will therefore have an incentive to attract patients, so they will make sure that the service they offer is what their patients want. And in turn they will stimulate other NHS hospitals to respond to what people want locally. NHS Hospital Trusts will also be able to set the rates of pay of their own staff and, within annual financing limits, to borrow money to help them respond to patient demand.

Third: **to enable hospitals which best meet the needs and wishes of patients to get the money to do so, the money required to treat patients will be able to cross administrative boundaries.** All NHS hospitals, whether run by health authorities or self-governing, will be free to offer their services to different health authorities and to the private sector. Consequently, a health authority will be better able to discharge its duty to use its available funds to secure a comprehensive service, including emergency services, by obtaining the best service it can whether from its own hospitals, from another authority's hospitals, from NHS Hospital Trusts or from the private sector.

Fourth: **to reduce waiting times and improve the quality of service, to help give individual patients appointment times they can rely on, and to help cut the long hours worked by some junior doctors, 100 new consultant posts will be created over the next three years.** This is in line with the number of fully trained doctors ready for consultant appointments in the relevant specialties. The new posts will be additional to the two per cent annual expansion of consultant numbers already planned.

Fifth: **to help the family doctor improve his service to patients, large GP practices will be able to apply for their own budgets to obtain a defined range of services direct from hospitals.** Again, in the interests of a better service to the patient, GPs will be encouraged to compete for patients by offering better services. And it will be easier for patients to choose (and change) their own GP as they wish.

Sixth: **to improve the effectiveness of NHS management, regional, district and family practitioner management bodies will be reduced in size and reformed on business lines, with executive and non-executive directors.** The Government believes that, in the interests of patients and staff, the era in which a £26 billion NHS is run by authorities which are neither truly representative nor fully management bodies must be ended. The confusion of roles will be replaced by clear remit and accountability.

Seventh: **to ensure that all concerned with delivering services to the patient make the best use of the resources available to them, quality of service and value for money will be more rigorously audited.** Arrangements for what doctors call "medical audit" will be extended throughout the Health Service, helping to ensure that the best quality of medical care is given to patients. The Audit Commission will assume responsibility for auditing the accounts of health authorities and other NHS bodies, and will undertake wide-ranging value for money studies. [. . .]

Public and private sectors working together

1.18 The NHS and the independent health sector should be able to learn from each other, to support each other and to provide services for each other. Anyone needing treatment can only benefit from such a development. People who choose to buy health care outside the Health Service benefit the community by taking pressure off the Service and add to the diversity of provision and choice. The Government expects to see further increases in the number of people wishing to make private provision for health care, but at the moment many people who do so during their working life find the cost of higher premiums difficult to meet in retirement. The Government therefore proposes to make it easier for people in retirement by allowing income tax relief on their private medical insurance premiums, whether paid by them or, for example, by their families on their behalf.

5 Everyone a private patient*

David Green

Attempting both to finance and supply health-care services through the NHS has given rise to two fundamental problems: endemic underfunding and inadequate competition.

Reliance on taxation has caused endemic underfunding

There is widespread attachment to the NHS on ethical grounds because access to medical care is ranked with food, clothing and shelter as one of the essentials which everyone should enjoy in a civilised society, regardless of ability to pay. And most people support the NHS because they believe it guarantees them access to health-care services when they fall ill. It is increasingly being recognised, however, that in practice the NHS is not always there when it is needed. Some say the solution is for the government to give more money to the NHS, but in Chapter 1 I will suggest that this remedy will bring only temporary relief because the NHS has a serious structural flaw, namely, that it lacks any link between demand and budgetary allocation. So long as health services are supplied free at the time of use and financed out of taxes, governments will always find themselves confronting not priced demand but unpriced expectations, uninhibited by contemplation of the other goods and services, like housing and education, which might have been enjoyed instead. [. . .]

If we truly want each citizen to enjoy guaranteed access to a well-defined set of essential health-care services, regardless of their ability to pay, then this objective could be more effectively accomplished if each person had a contract of insurance setting out his or her entitlements. But such a contract can be offered only if the actuarially sound insurance premium has been paid, whether wholly by the patient or, if poor, for him or her by the state. It goes without saying that the government must continue to fund health care for the poor to an acceptable standard. [. . .]

*This is an abridged extract from Green, D. (1988) *Everyone A Private Patient: An Analysis of the Structural Flaws in the NHS and How They Could be Remedied*, Institute of Economic Affairs, pp. 1–6, 81–3, 88–9.

Tax finance impedes competition and obstructs human ingenuity

The NHS has also impeded competition. The vast majority of people have only so much disposable income and because they are forced to pay for the monopolistic NHS they are not able to choose alternative provision. The absence of competition encourages bad service, as the government itself recognises; and, no less important, it discourages innovation and diversity.

A recurring theme throughout the study will be that there is virtue in diversity. American health care does not offer a ready-made blueprint, and this is still more obvious of the continental national insurance schemes. It does not matter where you look in the world, there is no obvious right answer. Problems remain and perverse incentives persist whether hospitals are paid a daily rate, or per case or unit of service, or are required to live within a global budget set by government; or whether doctors are paid a salary, capitation fee, fee per item of service, or per case. The conclusion I draw is that there is no point in searching for a single 'correct' solution. On the contrary, there is merit in variety.

A competitive market allows many ideas to be tried out at once, creating growing room for human ingenuity, so that if one answer does not work well there will always be something to compare it with, and alternatives to which consumers can turn for better service. Because it is a monopoly, the NHS not only denies people access to alternatives, but also conceals from them the information required to form a rational judgement about the quality of service they are getting. Greater competition affects:

(i)   the *providers* which enter the market – helping to ensure that those which prosper are the ones that satisfy consumers;
(ii) the *products/services* which are offered – those least attractive to consumers in terms of quality or performance tend to get eliminated; and
(iii) the *prices* at which services are sold – generally it encourages lower prices.

It must also be recognised that competition may produce perverse incentives and outcomes. [. . .]

Personal responsibility undermined

Perhaps the most damaging effect of the NHS promise of 'free' health care has been the way it has undermined the capacity of people for self-direction, and spread a child-like dependency on the state. The deception involved in compelling people to pay for a monopoly service whilst at the same time presenting that service as a kind of gift from government has been part and parcel of the welfare state since its early origins before the First World War, when Lloyd George used the specious slogan 'ninepence for fourpence' to encourage support for the 1911 National Insurance Act. Male contributions were fourpence, employers threepence and the government twopence, and people were encouraged to think of the additional fivepence as a gift. But a tax on employers is a tax on jobs, and governments do not have any money of their own, only other people's. Personal payment cannot be escaped, but we can choose whether the payment takes the *form* of a tax or a freely-paid price. Paying a price is a *disposal* of income, whereas a tax is a *deduction from* income which takes away personal responsibility for deciding how much money will go into health care and curtails personal responsibility for selecting the best arrangements for the supply of medical services.

Dependency also has wider, less tangible effects. In recent years the reforming spirit of the Government has been dominated by the necessity to face the economic facts of life. This was essential, but a civilised society cannot be built on economic policy alone. And if the recent economic revival is to be more than a respite from the post-war decades of decline we must seek to bring about a deeper rejuvenation of the cultural heritage that once meant that British ideas were admired throughout the world. The foundation stone of this culture was a spirit of self-direction. Parents freely accepted an obligation to provide for the important requirements of their children, including health care and education, and to raise them as good citizens. All but a minority of criminals and ne'er-do-wells freely accepted that right conduct was a personal duty to be fulfilled even when no one else was looking. But this independent spirit has been eroded by the welfare state ethic which said, not as collectivists insist, that people should help the unfortunate (an obligation in any event willingly accepted in Britain for centuries), but rather that everyone was a victim of circumstance, or 'the system'. And because we were all considered to be products of the environment all important services were to be provided by the state.

Ultimately this dependence on government undermines the chief foundation of a free society, the willingness of people freely to restrain their own exercise of freedom so that others may also enjoy it. [. . .]

Inclusion of the poor

One of the main arguments used against promoting personal choice is that a two-tier system will result. If the government funds health-care services for the poor but not for everyone then, so the argument runs, the poor will receive a poor quality service whilst people who can afford more will get superior care. Therefore, according to this line of reasoning, the government should finance health care for everyone and provide an equal service for them all. Some go so far as to advocate the abolition of the private sector to prevent the better-off buying extra services. The latter view has not carried much weight in recent years, largely because most people feel that if they want to go private they should be free to do so.

However, the idea that the government should finance health care from taxation in order that everyone can obtain 'equal' service is still powerful. It has been the dominant philosophy for the last 40 years and, as I have argued, it has failed because, among other things, it is based on the mistaken view that all health care is like emergency care and that consequently it should be free. But more important still, despite the rhetoric about equality, everyone is not treated equally by the NHS. If you work in the NHS, or you are a VIP, or you 'know the ropes', then it will almost certainly be possible to gain privileged service for yourself. In getting good service from the NHS, 'middle-class know-how' is of more value than 'middle-class money'.

In a competitive market, however, the dissatisfied customer can go to another hospital, and this very freedom to go elsewhere makes it more likely that providers will take the trouble to please their customers. Moreover, the comparisons and rivalry, which are the essence of competition, make it more likely that the dissatisfied customer will produce a general supply response which benefits many others. Above all, the simple freedom to go to an alternative provider requires no special aptitudes and therefore aids those with few social skills as much as the articulate and educated. In the absence of competition, complaints by the ordinary citizen may be ignored or even punished.

To sum up: the NHS does not provide equal treatment for all. Nor could it. In practice it puts everyone in a weaker position than they would be if they were personally responsible for their own health care. The poor are supposed to enjoy the same rights of access to medical care as everyone else, but in the first place, access depends partly on social skills and the poor disproportionately lack these skills. And in the second, they have no enforceable *rights*, as the two recent court cases fought by the distraught parents of the Birmingham hole-in-the-heart babies revealed. If, however, the government delineated a package of health-care services which it considered to be the civilised minimum, put a price on this package, and gave the poor sufficient money in the form of a voucher to buy it, the poor would be better off. They would have a clear entitlement to a well-defined set of services which was bought-and-paid-for and enforceable at law.

Much depends, of course, on how comprehensive a set of services is to be covered under the government package. There is a continuing need for debate about the standard of care government should provide the poor and how it should be adjusted over time. Should it, for instance, try to define the package in terms of the seriousness of the patient's ill-health? Should waiting times be built in for non-urgent surgery? Should it be linked to the services which the NHS is supposed (but fails in practice) to provide? In the latter case, it would not include private rooms, private telephones, 'cordon-bleu' food and the generally higher amenities available in private hospitals; nor would it include cosmetic surgery or a right of access to experimental techniques until they were tried and tested, but otherwise it would make available all the usual clinical services. [. . .]

Conclusion

The evidence from 40 years' experience of public *production* and *finance* through the NHS suggests that government should not attempt both to finance and produce health-care services. Instead, it should *finance* health care for those in need, to ensure that everyone has the power to buy health insurance cover, but it should not attempt to pay for all health-care services from taxation; it should *regulate*, by which I mean it should elaborate, refine, make and enforce the rules which enable a competitive market to serve the interests of all, rich and poor alike; and it should *publish* to enable people to make more effective choices.

Summary of policy proposals

- The NHS should be left intact, though pilot schemes to improve efficiency should be attempted.
- People dissatisfied with the NHS should be allowed to escape and to claim an age-weighted voucher representing the tax they had paid towards the NHS.
- They would be required to relinquish their claim to free NHS services and to take out private insurance to the value of the voucher or more, including catastrophe cover.
- Privately insured individuals or families could receive care, including emergency treatment, from the NHS as paying customers and would not be confined to using private hospitals.
- Separate vouchers would be available for hospital care (excluding long-stay) and primary care.
- The poor would receive a voucher sufficient to buy a specified set of health-care services.
- People opting out would take their voucher not direct to an insurance company but to a health purchase union, which would be responsible for making available several choices of insurance company.
- Most people will obtain cover through their employer or a private association, but in addition statutory health purchase unions independent of government would be established ultimately in each region (though initially only in each country of the UK).
- Insurance companies would be free to recruit individual subscribers, but they would not receive voucher payments unless the individual subscribed via a health purchase union.

6 Supporting families*

Home Office

Families are at the heart of our society. Most of us live in families and we value them because they provide love, support and care. They educate us, and they teach right from wrong. Our future depends on their success in bringing up children. That is why we are committed to strengthening family life.

There is now widespread recognition that a new approach supporting to the family is needed. Families are under stress. The divorce rate has risen sharply. There are more children being brought up in single parent households, and there is more child poverty, often as a direct consequence of family breakdown. Rising crime and drug abuse are indirect symptoms of problems in the family.

Saying that families are a good thing is not enough. Good intentions need to be carried through in practice.

But governments have to be wary about intervening in areas of private life and intimate emotion. We in Government need to approach family policy with a strong dose of humility. We must not preach and we must not give the impression that members of the Government are any better than the rest of the population in meeting the challenge of family life. They are not.

We also need to acknowledge just how much families have changed. Family structure has become more complicated, with many more children living with step-parents or in single parent households. They may face extra difficulties and we have designed practical support with these parents in mind. Women increasingly want to work and have careers as well as being mothers. Many fathers want more involvement with their children's upbringing.

A modern family policy needs to recognise these new realities. It also needs to be founded on clear principles.

First, the interests of children must be paramount. The Government's interest in family policy is primarily an interest in ensuring that the next generation gets the best possible start in life.

Second, children need stability and security. Many lone parents and unmarried couples raise their children every bit as successfully as married parents.

*This is an abridged extract from Home Office (1998) *Supporting Families – A Consultation Document*, The Stationery Office, pp. 4–6, 40–4.

But marriage is still the surest foundation for raising children and remains the choice of the majority of people in Britain. We want to strengthen the institution of marriage to help more marriages to succeed.

Third, wherever possible, government should offer support to all parents so that they can better support children, rather than trying to substitute for parents. There needs to be a clear understanding of the rights and responsibilities which fall to families and to government. Parents raise children, and that is how things should remain. More direct intervention should only occur in extreme circumstances, for example in cases of domestic violence or where the welfare of children is at stake.

Supporting families

Families depend on government for services such as education, health, social services, and law and order. In almost everything that government does, we can help families, neglect them or even do them active harm. So it must be right for government to have a policy towards the family, to provide the best support that we can.

This positive, supporting role is needed now more than ever. And just as the strains on families have increased over the years, so the support provided to help families needs to change too. Neither a 'back to basics' fundamentalism, trying to turn back the clock, nor an 'anything goes' liberalism which denies the fact that how families behave affects us all, is credible any more.

Instead, our approach concentrates on five areas where government can make a difference:

- ensuring that all parents have access to the advice and support they need, improving services and strengthening the ways in which the wider family and communities support and nurture family life
- improving family prosperity, reducing child poverty, and ensuring that the tax and benefit system properly acknowledges the costs of bringing up children
- making it easier for parents to spend more time with their children by helping families to balance work and home
- strengthening marriage and reducing the risks of family breakdown
- tackling the more serious problems of family life, including domestic violence and school-age pregnancy. [. . .]

Good parenting benefits us all. It provides children with the best possible start in life. It improves their health, schooling and prospects in later life, and it reduces the risk of serious social problems such as truancy, offending, and drug misuse.

All parents need support with their children's health, education and welfare, and many also want advice and guidance on how to bring up their children. However, parents do not want lectures from the state, or to be nagged or nannied. Except in exceptional circumstances, where the well-being of family members is at stake, it must be the decision of the parents when to ask for help or advice. Our priority is to provide better support for parents so that parents can provide better support for their children. [. . .]

All families face pressure in their everyday life and all families want some measure of support. But a small proportion of families encounter more serious problems and need particular help and assistance. We must not ignore their needs.

A modern family policy must be based on a realistic picture of the more severe pressures facing families today. Too many children live in poverty. Poor housing, social exclusion and lack of opportunity are at the root of many serious family problems. Every year thousands of families in difficulty receive help from Social Services Departments and voluntary organisations. Our broader strategies on social exclusion address these serious underlying problems. In a minority of families there are more acute problems such as youth offending, teenage pregnancy, domestic violence and problems with children's education which also need action. [. . .]

Problems with children's learning

Truancy and exclusions

In May 1998, the Government published the Social Exclusion Unit's report on truancy and exclusions from school. The report set out a framework for action involving a partnership between parents, communities, the police and social services as well as pupils and schools. In September 1998, exclusions had risen to 12,700. On 1 October 1998 the Government announced a new £500 million programme to cut truancy, unruly classroom behaviour and unnecessary exclusions. The target of the Government's strategy is to reduce truancy and unnecessary exclusion by one third by 2002. The new three year programme will involve close co-operation between parents, schools and the police with more home–school liaison, mentoring for difficult pupils and extra staff to follow up non-attendance with parents.

Home–school agreements

A reduction in truancy and exclusion can be achieved only in partnership with parents. Parents have a responsibility to work with their children's school to raise achievement and to take action to combat truancy and unacceptable behaviour. Parents can work more effectively with the school if they know what the school is trying to achieve and how they can help. We are therefore using the School Standards and Framework Act to introduce home–school agreements in all schools.

From September 1999, all schools will be required to have a written home–school agreement drawn up in consultation with parents. The agreement will explain the responsibilities of the school and of parents, and what the school expects of its pupils. Parents of pupils of compulsory school age will be asked to sign a declaration in support of the agreement. All agreements will set out the standard of education the school will provide; the ethos of the school; the need for regular and punctual attendance; discipline; homework; and the information which schools and parents will give one another. [. . .]

Youth offending

Children who grow up in stable, successful families are less likely to become involved in offending. Helping parents to exercise effective care and supervision of their young children can achieve long-term benefits by reducing the risk that children will become involved in delinquent or offending behaviour.

The Government has introduced several key measures in the Crime and Disorder Act 1998 to tackle juvenile offending, in part to speed up the time between arrest and sentencing to bring the crime home to offenders sooner; but also through initiatives to bring together everyone – particularly parents and local agencies – who can help young people avoid crime altogether, or reform their behaviour. These include **parenting orders, child safety orders, local child curfews and final warnings**. [. . .]

Parenting order

Some parents need support and direction in fulfilling their responsibilities and in helping prevent a child or young person from turning to crime. To help provide that support and direction, the Crime and Disorder Act provides for new powers for courts to impose a parenting order where a child or young person has been convicted of an offence.

The parenting order will help parents to change offending behaviour by their children. The order is intended to be used where the court is satisfied that action by one or both parents, through a parenting order, will help to prevent the child or young person from committing further offences. The order will include a requirement that parents attend counselling and guidance sessions where they will receive help in dealing with their children, for example to help parents to set and enforce consistent standards of behaviour from the young person.

The court may also impose a requirement to exercise control over a child's behaviour where firmer direction to the parents is judged to be necessary and appropriate. For example, the parent could be required to ensure that the child is home between certain hours or ensure that he or she is escorted to and from school by a responsible adult.

Child safety order

The Crime and Disorder Act also includes a number of new powers for the courts and the police to intervene more effectively at an early stage when a child is at risk of offending or first commits an offence. It provides for a child safety order which will be available in a Family Proceedings Court to protect children under 10 who are at risk of developing offending behaviour because of a lack of supervision or inappropriate activities or associations. The child will be supervised by a responsible officer, usually a local authority social worker. The order may impose requirements such as that the child should be at home a specified time or that they should stay away from specified places or people; and it may prohibit specified conduct, including truanting from school. The responsible officer will work closely with the child's parent in supervising the order and the court may also impose a parenting order on the parent when they impose a child safety order.

Local child curfews

Parents sometimes need help to enforce discipline. The local child curfew is intended to restore sensible standards in an area where children aged under 10 are allowed to stay out very late at night or in the early hours. They can be a nuisance, may be at risk, can be drawn into antisocial activity and are ruining their own life chances in the process. The local child curfew will support parents and the community in ending this problem and setting standards for the children.

Final warnings

If, despite the efforts of their parents, children and young people offend, they will come into contact with the police sooner or later. The final warning scheme, introduced by the Crime and Disorder Act 1998, replaces repeat cautioning and ensures that positive action will be taken in partnership with parents to address offending behaviour. The police will be able to call on new multi-agency youth offending teams to help parents to provide firm guidance on what is acceptable behaviour. Young offenders who receive a final warning will normally be expected to participate in a programme of constructive activities to address the causes of their behaviour and so to prevent reoffending. Where the parents of young offenders need support, these programmes can also include parenting classes.

7 The new NHS*

Secretary of State for Health

The third way

In paving the way for the new NHS the Government is committed to building on what has worked, but discarding what has failed. There will be no return to the old centralised command and control systems of the 1970s. That approach stifled innovation and put the needs of institutions ahead of the needs of patients. But nor will there be a continuation of the divisive internal market system of the 1990s. That approach which was intended to make the NHS more efficient ended up fragmenting decision-making and distorting incentives to such an extent that unfairness and bureaucracy became its defining features.

Instead there will be a 'third way' of running the NHS – a system based on partnership and driven by performance. It will go with the grain of recent efforts by NHS staff to overcome the obstacles of the internal market. Increasingly those working in primary care, NHS Trusts and Health Authorities have tried to move away from outright competition towards a more collaborative approach. Inevitably, however, these efforts have been only partially successful and their benefits have not as yet been extended to patients in all parts of the country.

This White Paper will put that right. It builds on the extensive discussions we have held with a wide range of NHS staff and organisations. It will develop this more collaborative approach into a new system for the whole NHS. It will neither be the model from the late 1970s nor the model from the early 1990s. It will be a new model for a new century.

Six key principles

Six important principles underlie the changes we are now proposing:

- first, to renew the NHS as a genuinely **national** service. Patients will get fair access to consistently high quality, prompt and accessible services right across the country

*This is an abridged extract from Secretary of State for Health (1997) *The New NHS – Modern, Dependable*, Cm. 3807, The Stationery Office, pp. 10–14, 17–18, 22–3.

- but second, to make the delivery of healthcare against these new national standards a matter of **local** responsibility. Local doctors and nurses who are in the best position to know what patients need will be in the driving seat in shaping services
- third, to get the NHS to work in **partnership**. By breaking down organisational barriers and forging stronger links with Local Authorities, the needs of the patient will be put at the centre of the care process
- but fourth, to drive **efficiency** through a more rigorous approach to performance and by cutting bureaucracy, so that every pound in the NHS is spent to maximise the care for patients
- fifth, to shift the focus onto quality of care so that **excellence** is guaranteed to all patients, and quality becomes the driving force for decision-making at every level of the service
- and sixth, to rebuild **public confidence** in the NHS as a public service, accountable to patients, open to the public and shaped by their views.

Keeping what works

There are some sound foundations on which the new NHS can be built. Not everything about the old system was bad. This Government believes that what counts is what works. If something is working effectively then it should not be discarded purely for the sake of it. The new system will go with the grain of the best of these developments.

The Government will retain the **separation between the planning of hospital care and its provision**. This is the best way to put into practice the new emphasis on improving health and on meeting the healthcare needs of the whole community. By empowering local doctors, nurses and Health Authorities to plan services we will ensure that the local NHS is built around the needs of patients. Hospitals and other agencies providing services will have a hand in shaping those plans but their primary duty will be to meet patients' requirements for high quality and easily accessible services. The needs of patients not the needs of institutions will be at the heart of the new NHS.

The Government will also build on the increasingly **important role of primary care** in the NHS. Most of the contact that patients have with the NHS is through a primary care professional such as a community nurse or a family doctor. They are best placed to understand their patients' needs as a whole and to identify ways of making local services more responsive. Family doctors who have been involved in commissioning services (either as fund-holders, or through multifunds, locality commissioning or the total purchasing model) have welcomed the chance to influence the use of resources to improve patient care. The Government wishes to build on these approaches, ensuring that all patients, rather than just some, are able to benefit.

Finally, the Government recognises the intrinsic strength of **decentralising responsibility for operational management**. By giving NHS Trusts control over key decisions they can improve local services for patients. The Government will build on this principle and let NHS Trusts help shape the locally agreed framework which will determine how NHS services develop. In the future the approach will be interdependence rather than independence.

Discarding what has failed

The internal market was a misconceived attempt to tackle the pressures facing the NHS. It has been an obstacle to the necessary modernisation of the health service. It created more problems than it solved. That is why the Government is abolishing it.

Ending fragmentation

The internal market split responsibility for planning, funding and delivering healthcare between 100 Health Authorities, around 3,500 GP fundholders (representing half of GP practices) and over 400 NHS Trusts. There was little strategic coordination. A fragmented NHS has been poorly placed to tackle the crucial issue of better integration across health and social care. People with multiple needs have found themselves passed from pillar to post inside a system in which individual organisations were forced to work to their own agendas rather than the needs of individual patients.

To overcome this fragmentation, in the new NHS all those charged with planning and providing health and social care services for patients will work to a jointly agreed local Health Improvement Programme. This will govern the actions of all the parts of the local NHS to ensure consistency and coordination. It will also make clear the responsibilities of the NHS and local authorities for working together to improve health.

Ending unfairness

The internal market created competition for patients. In the process it created unfairness for patients. Some family doctors were able to get a better deal for their patients, for financial rather than clinical reasons. Staff morale has been eroded by an emphasis on competitive values, at odds with the ethos of fairness that is intrinsic to the NHS and its professions. Hospital clinicians have felt disempowered as they have been deliberately pitted against each other and against primary care. The family doctor community has been divided in two, almost equally split between GP fundholders and non-fund-holders.

In the new NHS patients will be treated according to need and need alone. Cooperation will replace competition. GPs and community nurses will work together in the Primary Care Groups. Hospital clinicians will have a say in developing local Health Improvement Programmes.

Ending distortion

The market forced NHS organisations to compete against each other even when it would have made better sense to cooperate. Some were unwilling to share best practice that might benefit a wider range of patients in case they forfeited competitive advantage. Quality has been at best variable.

In the new NHS, there will be new mechanisms to share best practice so that it becomes available to patients wherever they live. A new national performance framework for ensuring high performance and quality will, over time, tackle variable standards of service. [. . .]

Driving quality

The new NHS will have quality at its heart. Without it there is unfairness. Every patient who is treated in the NHS wants to know that they can rely on receiving high quality care when they need it. Every part of the NHS, and everyone who works in it, should take responsibility for working to improve quality. This must be quality in its broadest sense: doing the right things, at the right time, for the right people, and doing them right – first time. And it must be the quality of the patient's experience as well as the clinical result – quality measured in terms of prompt access, good relationships and efficient administration.

There is much to build on. Clearing away the distraction of the market will help staff get attention back where it counts. But new and systematic action is needed, to raise standards and ensure consistency. There have been some serious lapses in quality. When they have occurred they have harmed individual patients and dented public confidence.

This White Paper sets out three areas for action to drive quality into all parts of the NHS: **national standards and guidelines** for services and treatments; **local measures** to enable NHS staff to take responsibility for improving quality; and a new **organisation to address shortcomings**.

Nationally there will be:

- new evidence-based **National Service Frameworks** to ensure consistent access to services and quality of care right across the country
- a new **National Institute for Clinical Excellence** to give a strong lead on clinical and cost-effectiveness, drawing up new guidelines and ensuring they reach all parts of the health service.

Locally there will be:

- teams of **local GPs and community nurses** working together in new Primary Care Groups to shape services for patients, concentrating on the things which really count – prompt, accessible, seamless care delivered to a high standard
- explicit quality standards in local **service agreements** between Health Authorities, Primary Care Groups and NHS Trusts, reflecting national standards and targets

- a new system of **clinical governance** in NHS Trusts and primary care to ensure that clinical standards are met, and that processes are in place to ensure continuous improvement, backed by a new **statutory duty** for quality in NHS Trusts.

A new **Commission for Health Improvement** will be established to support and oversee the quality of clinical services at local level, and to tackle shortcomings. It will be able to intervene where necessary. The Secretary of State will also have reserve powers to intervene directly when a problem has not been gripped. [. . .]

Roles and responsibilities

The new NHS will mean new roles and responsibilities for Health Authorities, NHS Trusts and the Department of Health. Primary Care Groups will also be developed across the country.

Health Authorities will be leaner bodies with stronger powers to improve the health of their residents and oversee the effectiveness of the NHS locally. Over time, they will relinquish direct commissioning functions to Primary Care Groups. Working with local authorities, NHS Trusts and Primary Care Groups, they will take the lead in drawing up three-year Health Improvement Programmes which will provide the framework within which all local NHS bodies will operate. These will be backed by a new duty of partnership. Health Authorities will allocate funds to Primary Care Groups on an equitable basis, and hold them to account. Links with social services will be strengthened. Fewer Health Authorities covering larger areas will emerge as a product of these changes, flowing from local discussion rather than national edict.

Primary Care Groups comprising all GPs in an area together with community nurses will take responsibility for commissioning services for the local community. This will not affect the independent contractor status of GPs. The new Primary Care Groups will replace existing commissioning and fund-holding arrangements. All Primary Care Groups will be accountable to Health Authorities, but will have freedom to make decisions about how they deploy their resources within the framework of the Health Improvement Programme. Over time, Primary Care Groups will have the opportunity to become freestanding Primary Care Trusts.

NHS Trusts, the bodies that provide patient services in hospitals and in the community, will be party to the local Health Improvement Programme and will agree long term service agreements with Primary Care Groups. These service agreements will generally be organised around a particular care group (such as children) or disease area (such as heart disease) linked to the new National Service Frameworks. In this way, hospital clinicians will be able to make a more significant contribution to service planning. National model agreements will be developed. NHS Trusts will have a statutory duty for quality.

The **Department of Health,** and within it the NHS Executive, will shoulder responsibility for action genuinely needed at a national level. It will integrate health and social services policy to give a national lead which others will be expected to follow locally. It will also work with the clinical professions to develop National Service Frameworks, linked to national action to implement them across the NHS. For the first time, there will be an annual national survey to allow systematic comparisons of the experience of patients and their carers over time, and between different parts of the country. A new NHS Charter will set out new rights and responsibilities for patients. The Secretary of State will have reserve powers to intervene where Health Authorities, Primary Care Groups and NHS Trusts are failing.

8 Saving lives*

Secretary of State for Health

England is a rich country – rich in its people, rich in its resources, rich in innovation, rich in its values, rich in its history, rich in its future. Yet in this rich country, not everyone has an equal chance of healthy life. Too many people suffer from poor health. Too many people are ill for much of their lives. Too many people die too young from preventable diseases.

Saving Lives: Our Healthier Nation is an action plan for tackling poor health and improving the health of everyone in England, especially the worst off.

We believe that if we can achieve the bold objectives we are setting we have the opportunity of savings as many as 300,000 lives over the next 10 years.

But to do that, we have to tackle the four main killers – the illnesses which, together with accidents, play the greatest part in causing preventable deaths and ill-health: cancer, coronary heart disease and stroke and mental illness. Together they account for more than 75 per cent of all the people who die before the age of 75 years. Combating these killers will not end them: they will still cut into people's lives and the lives of their families. But we can reduce their impact.

So we are setting new, tougher and challenging targets in each of these priority areas. By 2010:

- Cancer
  to reduce the death rate from cancer in people under 75 by at least a fifth – saving 100,000 lives

- Coronary heart disease and stroke
  to reduce the death rate from coronary heart disease and stroke and related diseases in people under 75 by at least two fifths – saving 200,000 lives

- Accidents
  to reduce the death rate from accidents by at least a fifth and to reduce the rate of serious injury from accidents by at least a tenth – saving 12,000 lives

*This is an abridged extract from Secretary of State for Health (1999) *Saving Lives: Our Healthier Nation*, Cm. 4386, The Stationery Office, pp. 1–2, 5–10.

- Mental health
  to reduce the death rate from suicide and undetermined injury by at least
  a fifth – saving 4,000 lives [. . .]

Our modern approach is reflected in the goals of this White Paper:

- to improve the health of the population as a whole by increasing the
  length of people's lives and the number of years people spend free from
  illness; and
- to improve the health of the worst off in society and to narrow the health
  gap.

Our twin goals are consistent with the health strategies being adopted by
the other countries of the United Kingdom. They are also consistent with the
World Health Organisation (Europe)'s new programme for the 21st Century
Health 21 and the European Community's developing strategy for public
health.

We propose the first comprehensive Government plan focused on the main
killers of people in our country. We are determined to succeed in our goals –
and if we do, then by cutting needless early deaths from cancer, coronary heart
disease and stroke, accidents and suicide, there is the real prospect of reducing
the number of deaths from these causes by up to 300,000 by the year 2010.

This is a bold ambition. Improving health for all and tackling health
inequality is a challenging objective – a crusade for health on a scale never
undertaken by Government before. We will measure the success of our
ambition by the numbers of lives saved, and by the improvement in the health
of the people of our country. The task is clear: to give everyone in our nation,
whatever their background, the chance to lead a long and healthy life.

The way to better health

Improving health means tackling the causes of poor health. We know that the
causes of ill-health are many: a complex interaction between personal, social,
economic and environmental factors.

In our new approach to better health, we want to break with the past. We
want to move beyond the old arguments and tired debates which have
characterised so much consideration of public health issues, including those
who say that nothing can be done to improve the health of the poorest, and
those who say that individuals are solely to blame for their own ill-health.

These arguments have focused not on what can be achieved, but on what
role there is for those involved – including whether there is a role for Government, or whether these matters are solely issues of personal responsibility.

We reject the polarity of these positions. We refuse to accept that there is
no role for anything other than the personal. Equally we refuse to accept that
for some people poor health is inevitable.

We reject that hopelessness. As with our policies on education and employment, we reject the inevitability of wasted lives and wasted generations – the

belief that nothing can be done. As with education and employment, we believe that people can be instrumental in shaping their own futures, rather than being victims of them. And there is a clear role for local agencies acting together, offering help with the decisions that individuals make.

People are responsible for their own actions in health as in other areas. But the decisions people take over their health are more likely to result in better health and a healthier life if they have the opportunity to make informed decisions.

Our new approach is rooted in precisely that balance. We believe that individuals can, should and do affect how healthy they are. But we believe too that there are powerful factors beyond the control of the individual which can harm health. The Government has a clear responsibility to address these fundamental problems. Striking a new balance – a third way – linking individual and wide action is at the heart of our new approach.

Smoking provides a striking example of these various factors at work. We have set out our policy on smoking in our White Paper on tobacco, *Smoking Kills*. Smoking is the most powerful factor which determines whether people live beyond middle age. And smoking more than any other identifiable factor contributes to the gap in healthy life expectancy between the most deprived and the most advantaged. But it is at the same time a factor about which individuals can make a decision. For many people who smoke, the decision to give up is not an easy one. Nicotine is addictive. But there is a clear route to better health. It is a clear route too which those who are more fortunate tend to take more than those who are less fortunate. We want people to stop smoking. But we also want that policy to have a greater impact among the less fortunate, where the harm caused by smoking is greater. To do that we have to address the complex interactions of social, economic and personal factors. Tackling smoking achieves both our objectives – improved health for all, and especially better health for the worse off.

For people to make such decisions against the background of such powerful determinants, they need to make informed decisions. Such decisions must be based on information about the risks involved in a range of activities, practices and products. People cannot and should not be pressured into responsibility. We do not believe in the old nanny-state approach. But there is a powerful role for Government in making clear the nature and scale of risk, and in some cases, taking protective action in the light of it.

We recognise that this is an unusual area for Government action. Governments can set the preconditions for success in improving health. But Governments alone cannot determine success. To do that, the Government needs to work in partnership with others.

A three-way partnership

Partnership is a key element of the Government's approach to a wide range of issues. Partnerships in areas such as business, education, crime prevention and many others are at the core of the way the Government carries out its work. Partnership is at the heart of our new approach to better health in *Saving Lives: Our Healthier Nation.*

To improve health and to tackle health inequality, we need a new three-way partnership, comprising:

- individuals
- communities
- Government

Individuals are central to our new vision for better health. People need to take responsibility for their own health – and many are doing so. There is a new and clear realisation that individuals can improve their health, by what they do and the actions they take.

Better health information – and the means of applying that information – is the bedrock on which improvements to the health of individuals will be made. But better health opportunities and decisions are not easily available to everyone. For example, membership of a gym may not be an option for someone in a poor neighbourhood or a single mother.

Communities working in partnership through local organisations are the best means of delivering the better information, better services and better community-wide programmes which will lead to better health. The roles of the NHS and of local authorities are crucial. They must become organisations for health improvement, as well as for health care and service provision. We are underlining this joint responsibility by the new duty of partnership on NHS bodies and local government in the Health Act. All aspects of the way that the NHS works with other local bodies, from the reorganisation of primary care services to the development of healthy neighbourhoods, from the *NHS Direct* phone-line to the creation of a new Health Development Agency, will be geared not just to treatment of illness but to the prevention and early detection of ill-health.

Initiatives including the *Healthy Citizens* programme, health improvement programmes and health action zones will all provide a local focus for the delivery of information and programmes at local level aimed at helping individuals improve their health and the health of their families. The dynamic of health improvement will for the first time be integrated into the local delivery of health care.

Government will play its part by creating the right conditions for individuals to make healthy decisions. Across a range of Government policy, we are focusing on the factors that increase the likelihood of poor health – poor housing, poverty, unemployment, crime, poor education and family breakdown.

The Government is taking action to combat social exclusion, to make work pay, to support children and families, to promote community safety – all moves which will do much to improve people's health, and to improve especially the health of the least fortunate in our country.

An integrated approach

This is our new contract for health. Our new approach, based on our three-way partnership between people, local communities and the Government, adopts a new way of tackling poor health which is both inclusive and integrated, comprehensive and coherent.

It ensures that all involved in improving health play their part. Individuals have the responsibility to improve their health, and the health of their families. Local agencies, led by health and local authorities, have the responsibility for delivering local services and local programmes which will enable people to claim the right of better health. And the Government has the responsibility of giving everyone throughout our country the opportunity for better education, better housing, and better prospects of securing work.

Common sense suggests that this integrated approach to tackling poor health is best. It is supported by the scientific and medical evidence. Reducing the impact of cancer and heart disease, for example, can be done only if we tackle smoking effectively. In turn, tackling smoking depends on relieving the conditions – social stress, unemployment, poor education, crime, vandalism – which lead far more people in disadvantaged communities to smoke than in other sections of the community.

Our approach, based on partnership between individuals, communities and Government, is not one which ranks action by one above the other: by emphasising integration our strategy will ensure that the whole will be greater than the sum of the parts.

9 A new universalism*

World Health Organisation

Health systems in some countries perform well. Others perform poorly. An accumulation of applied research efforts and practical experience now suggests some reasons for these differences. Countries differ, of course, and lessons that are useful to one country may have little value to others. Furthermore, evidence about what has worked – and what has not – constitutes only one of several factors influencing the decisions that shape health systems. That said, for many government officials, as for many clinicians, evidence *does* matter. But clearly, for national purposes, only national officials can judge the relevance and political feasibility of using evidence generated from other countries and other times. [. . .]

Before turning to the evidence, it is worth listing the goals of health systems – as WHO sees them. Goals can be phrased in many ways, and each goal may have different relevance in different contexts. Yet the following core list of goals for health system development is likely to elicit broad agreement:

- improving health status;
- reducing health inequalities;
- enhancing responsiveness to legitimate expectations;
- increasing efficiency;
- protecting individuals, families and communities from financial loss;
- enhancing fairness in the financing and delivery of health care.

This chapter also considers the following questions. How can the limits to government involvement and government finance be recognized, and how can choices be made that best achieve the right balance between systemic goals while recognizing budgetary and other limits? What incentives for providers of care will constrain cost escalation while motivating compassionate service of high quality? Independently of sources of finance, what are reasonable roles for private and public providers of care to play? How can research and development to underpin continued health improvement glob-

*This is an abridged extract from World Health Organisation (1999) *The World Health Report 1999 – Making a Difference*, WHO, pp. 31–3, 37, 39–43, 46.

ally be sustained in a context where most health finance is national? Finally, and most important, what is the role of government in financing health services? Analytic and empirical work provides no specific answers to these questions but, rather, assembles the evidence on consequences resulting from the choices made in different countries at different times. The accumulated evidence may, in some cases, suggest that certain policies have worked well, while others have worked poorly.

Where, to anticipate the findings of the chapter, do the values of WHO lead when combined with the available evidence? *They lead away from a form of universalism that has governments attempting to provide and finance everything for everybody.* This "classical" universalism, although seldom advanced in extreme form, shaped the formation of many European health systems. It achieved important successes. But classical universalism fails to recognize both resource limits and the limits of government.

The findings also lead away from market-oriented approaches that ration health services according to the ability to pay. Not only do market-oriented approaches to finance lead to intolerable inequity with respect to a fundamental human right, but growing bodies of theory and evidence indicate them to be inefficient as well. Market mechanisms have enormous utility in many sectors and have underpinned rapid economic growth for over a century in Europe and elsewhere. But the very countries that have relied heavily on market mechanisms to achieve the high incomes they enjoy today are the same countries that rely most heavily on governments to finance their health services. Therein lies a lesson. Health is an important component of national welfare. Achieving high health outcomes requires a combination of universal entitlement and tight control over expenditure.

This report advocates a "new universalism" that recognizes governments' limits but retains government responsibility for the leadership and finance of health systems. The new universalism welcomes diversity and, subject to appropriate guidelines, competition in the provision of services. At the same time it recognizes that if services are to be provided for all then not all services can be provided. The most cost-effective services in a given setting should be provided first. The new universalism recognizes private providers as an important source of care in many countries; welcomes private sector involvement in supplying service providers with drugs and equipment; and it encourages increased public and private investment in generating the new drugs, equipment and vaccines that will underpin long-term improvements in health. [. . .]

Renewing progress towards universal coverage

A clear historical lesson emerges from health systems development in the 20th century: spontaneous, unmanaged growth in any country's health system cannot be relied upon to ensure that the greatest health needs are met.[1,2] Public intervention is necessary to achieve universal access. In any country, the greatest burden of ill-health and the biggest risk of avoidable morbidity or mortality are borne by the poor. While progress towards universal access to health care of an acceptable quality has been substantial in this century, the distribution of services in most countries of the world remains highly skewed in favour of the better-off. While the equity arguments for universal public finance are widely accepted, what is less well known is that this approach achieves greater efficiency as well. [. . .]

Health care coverage

The two decades since the Alma-Ata Declaration have not seen the realization of the wished-for rapid and sustained progress towards universally accessible basic health care. The global picture is very uneven, with many countries dismantling their social protection mechanisms in health rather than expanding them. Major shifts in the 1990s in formerly socialist countries towards market economies have often been accompanied by a widespread movement of the health workforce into private practice, particularly in urban areas. In the decades up to the 1980s, many socialist countries had established universally accessible health care systems. Although these may have been inefficient, bureaucratic and unresponsive to patients' needs, basic care and, in many cases, secondary and tertiary care as well, was effectively prepaid and available to almost the entire population for little or no payment at the time of need. Most people in these countries have found that they have now to pay more – officially or unofficially – for their health care, and access to care is increasingly reflecting the ability to pay. In just a decade, China dismantled its Rural Cooperative Medical System, built up from the 1950s to provide health insurance protection for the great majority, and in the 1980s made some four-fifths of the total population uninsured, in other words fully responsible for their own health care costs. [. . .]

The industrialized countries have largely preserved their systems of near-universally accessible and prepaid health care, sometimes (as in Canada, New Zealand and the United Kingdom) implementing major organizational reform programmes. However, the fraction of the population under age 65 without private or public insurance protection in the United States has continued to grow, from nearly 15% in 1987 to nearly 18% in 1996.[3] And other countries have begun to shift payment responsibilities for long term care directly onto patients and their families. Inequality in health outcomes between the poorest and best-off groups have widened in many industrialized countries. [. . .]

Policy choices

Some, but by no means all, health policy choices involve trade-offs among the goals set out at the beginning of this chapter. As China's and Sri Lanka's experience in the 1950s and 1960s has shown, in situations of great poverty it is possible to make dramatic improvements in equitable access to care and simultaneously to bring about major improvements in health outcomes, while still keeping total public spending on health at modest levels. Canada's shift to national health insurance simultaneously achieved both better health and economic gains. Ensuring that poor people benefit from the promotive, preventive and curative interventions that are already available not only improves their access to health care, it substantially contributes to reducing the total burden of illness facing a region or a country. Opportunities now exist to make huge inroads into avoidable health problems, whilst cementing solidarity between different social strata.

To achieve this potential, the poorest and sickest people have to be reached by health promotion and prevention programmes, and they have to be able to get to clinics or health posts (private, public or nongovernment) where the right kind of treatment is available for common local, treatable conditions. And there must be no significant price barrier at the time poor people need services. Universal coverage means that, irrespective of the source of funds, the health care system functions like a national health insurance system, prepaid either through tax revenues or through employment-based social insurance, to ensure the largest possible pool of risks. There has to be a shift in the mentality of the system from funding the "needs" of the service delivery infrastructure to purchasing services according to the health care needs of the population. Instead of a series of independent and uncoordinated insurance and health financing schemes, each with its own beneficiaries, benefits and sometimes with its own set of health facilities and professionals, a national health insurance system means a merging of risk protection responsibilities into the largest possible pool, or coordination of the benefit packages financed from different funding sources, with the ultimate aim of funding a comprehensive set of covered services from the resources of a single fund. A single fund for the pooling of risks allows for many options in the way incentives are set for individual providers of care, including the option of shifting risk to providers. [. . .]

Recent comparative research, measuring equity in both the financing burden and the use of services by different income groups in countries, shows that the least organized and most inequitable way of paying for health care is on an out-of-pocket basis; people pay for their medical care when they need and use it. The financing burden falls disproportionally on the poorest (who face higher health care costs than the better-off), and the financial barrier means that use of services is lower among the lower income groups, in spite of their need being typically higher.[4]

The market response to a user-fee based system is through the development of private insurance. Insurers see a profitable opportunity. People prepay through insurance premiums, so that they do not have to live with unpredictably large health care bills. This method of financing entails some pooling of risks among the insured, but creates access inequities between the insured, who will get preferential access to better care, and the non-insured. Experience with commercial health insurance markets shows that they are both unstable and difficult to regulate, with each insurer constantly adjusting the risk profile of the beneficiary group in order to ensure that revenues are greater than expenditures. [. . .]

Most equitable of all in terms of the way the health financing burden is shared, and in allowing equal access to care for people with comparable need, are risk pooling systems based on tax revenue financing, such as in Canada, Cuba, Denmark, New Zealand, Norway, Spain, Sweden and the United Kingdom. The risk pool is the entire resident population, and the insurance function against the costs of health care is implemented by government, funded by taxes which, in a progressive system, take a larger share of income from the rich than from the poor. [. . .]

New universalism

To maximize the efficiency and equity gains, and create "win-win" situations in poorer countries with large burdens of illness, practical steps towards universal coverage need to be taken. There is no single blueprint available for replication by all countries. But a number of key design features for progress to a new universalism in health are now apparent.

*   *Membership is defined to include the entire population, i.e. it is compulsory.*
    Whether this is citizenship or residence, the purpose is to ensure that the population covered is defined inclusively.

*   *Universal coverage means coverage for all, not coverage of everything.*
    The prepayment system, financed by government, corporations and better-off individuals, will reflect a country's overall level of economic development. It will be a limited fund, not able to pay for all of those services that the population – and the health workforce – would like to see provided at no charge. Lower priority services, which will vary from one country to another, will only be available for payment. A benefit package has to be clearly defined in the light of the resources available and the cost of top priority health interventions, an assessment of the services and inputs for which individuals are able and willing to pay out of their own pockets, and the political feasibility of various choices.

*   *Provider payment is not made by the patient at the time he or she uses the health service.*
    Health care always has to be paid for. But the way it is paid for makes a major difference to who gets care and to overall levels of health. Out-of-pocket payments penalize the cash poor: those who work outside the cash economy, or who have only seasonal or occasional cash income, or who are unemployed. Heavy reliance on out-of-pocket payment sets the wrong incentives for both users and providers, and results in an inequitable financing burden and barriers to access for the poorest. Prepayment allows a wide range of incentive-setting methods for the efficient purchasing of services.

- *Services may be offered by providers of all types.*
  Provided that health practices and health facilities meet certain quality standards and that they are subject to similar levels of managerial flexibility, their ownership status should not matter. A stronger purchaser setting standard rates of remuneration and enforcing a common set of quality and utilization regulations will enable the most efficient provider of services to flourish. Such arrangements will allow the very large numbers of private providers, who are essentially the first points of contact with the health system in many low-income countries, to be brought within a structured but pluralistic health care system, benefiting from its resources and subject to sanction and regulation by professional and public bodies. [. . .]

To enable the whole population of even the richest country to have access to effective care of good quality, many choices have to be made. These choices concern health interventions, as well as the way these interventions are delivered through health systems. In both cases, choices should take account of research into effectiveness in order to ensure the development of an optimal strategy. An open and informed debate about priorities in health is also a necessary part of this strategy. Informing this debate is a critical task for research, and it is one being addressed by WHO's new Global Programme on Evidence. Unless these choices are made by responsible authorities, nationally and locally, and their implementation is monitored, service provision always tends to favour the better-off groups, both in terms of where services are available and what services are offered. The objectives enumerated at the beginning of this chapter are more likely to be achieved when appropriate political and financial mechanisms complement performance data in making authorities accountable to the populations they are meant to serve. To select key interventions and to orient health services towards entire populations combines universalism with economic realism. This "new universalism" is an attainable goal for the early years of the next century.

References

1 Arrow, K.J. Uncertainty and the welfare economics of medical care. *American economic review*, 1963, 53: 941–973.

2 Barr, N. *The economics of the welfare state. Second edition.* California, Stanford University Press, 1993.

3 Hoffman, C. *Uninsured in America: A chart book.* Washington DC, Kaiser Commission on Medicaid and the Uninsured, 1998.

4 Doorslaer, E., Wagstaff, A., Rutten, F. *Equity in the finance and delivery of health care: An international perspective.* Oxford, Oxford University Press, 1993.

Part II
Social stratification and health

Introduction

Over the half century of its existence, the NHS has found itself subject to the effects of different ideological forces and political agendas. On the threshold of the twenty-first century its commitment to ideals of social justice is being scrutinised and its principle of 'universalism' redefined. As welfare restructuring continues, the NHS now operates in an arena in which the relationships between various service providers is changing. A 'mixed economy' of welfare is now well established and the incorporation of the independent sector into the new 'welfare regime' that is emerging to replace the 'welfare state' continues to develop. Perhaps the most significant challenge facing the NHS in 2001 is the same as it faced in 1948, namely the existence of major inequalities in health within the British population. In this section of the reader the focus is on this major area of enquiry and debate in the sociology and politics of health.

The optimism of the immediate post-war welfare settlement, combined with the growing affluence of the late 1950s/early 1960s, was shattered by the 'rediscovery of poverty' in the mid-1960s by sociologists. This work is represented by an extract from Abel-Smith and Townsend's influential study from 1965 (Reading 10), which suggested that traditional social inequalities persisted in an apparent climate of plenty. Their work challenged two core assumptions which, they argued, continued to fuel discussion of social and economic policy in Britain after the Second World War, namely that poverty had been abolished and that Britain was a much more equal society.

In the field of health, social inequalities expressed themselves in many ways including unequal access to health care resources and facilities. Tudor Hart's 'inverse care law' (Tudor Hart 1971) suggested that those with the greatest need for health care actually received least. The inverse care law has persisted and, with it, growing inequalities in health have been well documented.

Two readings in the collection illustrate this growth in health inequalities: an extract from the seminal 'Black Report' from 1979 (Reading 11) and the 1994 article by Phillimore, Beattie and Townsend (Reading 12) which documents the widening gulf of health in northern England during the period 1981–91. 'Black' identified the pattern of health inequality in Britain that was seen to take on a number of 'distinctive forms', with gender, geographical location, race and ethnicity, and social class all existing as significant dimensions of inequality. Disturbingly, the report concluded that trends in health inequalities were continuing to deteriorate in Britain from the late 1940s. This deterioration in health during the period in which the 'welfare state' was established and consolidated has continued in the wake of 'Black' with political indifference to health inequalities guaranteeing their persistence in the 1990s. Some fifteen years after the Black Report's publication, Phillimore and collegues demonstrate widening mortality differentials between the most affluent and deprived areas in a region of northern England, and conclude that these mortality patterns are linked to 'material conditions rather than individual behaviour'.

In considering the social and environmental forces affecting health and access to health care, the significance of various dimensions and aspects of social stratification has been well documented, including 'ethnicity' (Smaje 1995), 'gender' (Doyal 1995) and 'social exclusion' (Purdy and Banks 1999). In the present collection a short extract from Doyal (Reading 13) describes the 'picture of health' experienced by women in both the developed and poorer countries of the world. Despite cultural variations in the concepts of sickness and health, and in the subjective experience of illness, women's physical and mental health is harmed in broadly similar ways. Inequalities in mortality and morbidity rates are shown to exist between women from different social groups and in the life expectancy of women in rich and poor nations. Doyal argues that Western medicine is limited in its ability to deal with many health problems experienced by women due to its separation of individuals from the 'social and cultural contexts of their lives' in which these health problems arise and develop.

Identifying inequalities in health has proved easier and more straightforward than explaining their existence. Explanations of inequality can be found in the ideological and political agendas which have informed health policy and public provision of services, agendas which have either chosen to ignore or address such inequalities. A significant example of the former has been the persistence of an 'ideology and politics of victim blaming' in which those sections of the population experiencing the poorest health and the greatest inequalities are effectively held to be responsible for their own poor health. This common strategy for explaining away health inequalities is the subject of Crawford's influential 1977 discussion of victim blaming (Reading 14). Crawford argues that the new victim blaming ideology of 'individual responsibility for health' which emerged in the United States in the 1970s served both to challenge and reorder the public's expectations regarding their right for access to medical services, and diverted attention from the social and economic causes of disease and ill-health in favour of emphasising the role of individual lifestyle choices. By encouraging individuals to avoid 'at risk' behaviours and change their lifestyles accordingly, the ideology of individual responsibility meets the demands of an economic imperative of cost curtailment by justifying reductions in entitlement to health services and by shifting the burden of medical costs onto users themselves. Such a strategy of victim blaming can only exacerbate existing inequalities in health and in access to health services (Purdy 1999).

Conflicting explanations for health inequalities can be usefully situated in relation to an ideology and politics of victim blaming. These include: (1) 'social selection' accounts (for example, West 1991) which emphasise the importance of processes of social mobility in accounting for the social class gradient in health. The higher and more affluent social classes are seen to collect the healthier members of each generation of the population and the poorer and lower social classes the least healthy members; (2) 'cultural/behavioural' approaches (for example, DOH 1992) which consider poor health to be largely the outcome of individuals engaging in unhealthy behaviour due to either ignorance or irrational/irresponsible choices, and which may suggest that certain communities are characterised by more unhealthy 'lifestyles' relative to others due to cultural or sub-cultural influences; and (3) 'materialist' or 'structural' explanations (for example, Blackburn 1991) which emphasise the role of social and economic forces, and conditions such as poverty, unemployment, housing and environmental pollution in generating poor health.

The complexities involved in adequately explaining health inequalities is illustrated in a recent overview (Reading 15) of the field since the 'Black Report' first proposed its materialist explanation. The extract produced here 'samples' the excellent *Sociology of Health & Illness* 1998 special issue on health inequalities, describing many promising developments in health inequalities research which simultaneously address questions of 'agency' and 'structure'. In particular, Bartley and colleagues note the emergence of a new 'lifecourse' perspective in the field, a perspective which 'encourages an attempt to embrace the complexity of social causation, rather than the production of simple but inadequate unitary explanations' (p. 565) and thereby address the 'fine grain' of the health gradient.

Just as explanations of health inequalities may reflect particular ideological and political preferences, so action that is proposed to tackle inequalities will endorse similar preferences: for example, calling on individuals to make healthier lifestyle choices rather than calling on central government to redistribute income. The range of possible actions to address and reduce inequalities in health is well illustrated by an extract taken from Sir Donald Acheson's recent independent review of inequalities in health commissioned by the New Labour government (Reading 16). Acheson argues that the evidence reviewed supports a socio-economic explanation of health inequalities according to which 'determinants of health' such as employment, education and income are recognised to be just as important as lifestyle factors. Consequently, policies to tackle inequalities in health need to be both 'upstream' (for example, focusing on generating employment opportunities) and 'downstream' (for example, offering assistance to help individuals to give up smoking) in scope. In this view, policies to reduce and eradicate inequalities in health are necessarily cross-departmental and the Acheson Report emphasises in the first of its recommendations the need for government to assess the impact on health inequalities of all policies which are likely to have an affect on health and to formulate such policies wherever possible to 'favour the less well off'. In total, Acheson makes thirty-nine recommendations, two general and thirty-seven covering the following policy areas and stages of the life course: poverty, income, tax and benefits; education; employment; housing and environment; mobility, transport and pollution; nutrition and the Common Agricultural Policy; mothers, children and families; young people and adults of working age; older people; ethnicity; gender; and the National Health Service. In the extract produced here the range and diversity of interventions recommended is illustrated by examples taken from a selection of these policy areas and age groups.

Whilst the Acheson Report has been welcomed for identifying policy options to tackle health inequalities rather than simply assembling more evidence of their existence (Labonte 1999), its failure to prioritise its recommendations and the interventions they advocate has been seen to be a significant weakness (Davey Smith *et al.* 1999). The adequacy of the government's response to Acheson (DOH 1999) has been questioned and renewed calls have been made on New Labour to redistribute income in order to effectively tackle inequalities in health (Townsend 1999; Shaw *et al.* 1999) in the face of new evidence of the continuing and deteriorating north–south divide since its election to office (Shaw *et al.* 1999).

References

Blackburn, C. (1991) *Poverty and Health: Working with Families*, Milton Keynes: Open University Press.

Davey Smith, G., Dorling, D., Gordon, D. and Shaw, M. (1999) 'The widening health gap: what are the solutions?', *Critical Public Health* 9: 151–70.

Department of Health (DOH) (1992) *The Health of the Nation: A Strategy for Health in England*, London: DOH.

Department of Health (DOH) (1999) *Reducing Health Inequalities: An Action Report*, London: DOH.

Doyal, L. (1995) *What Makes Women Sick: Gender and the Political Economy of Health*, London: Macmillan.

Labonte, R. (1999) 'Some comments on the Acheson Report', *Critical Public Health* 9: 171–4.

Purdy, M. (1999) 'The health of which nation? Health, social regulation and the new consensus', in M. Purdy and D. Banks (eds) *Health and Exclusion: Policy and Practice in Health Provision*, London: Routledge.

Purdy, M. and Banks, D. (eds) (1999) *Health and Exclusion: Policy and Practice in Health Provision*, London: Routledge.

Shaw, M., Dorling, D., Gordon, D. and Davey Smith, G. (eds) (1999) *The Widening Gap: Health Inequalities and Policy in Britain*, Bristol: The Policy Press.

Smaje, C. (1995) *Health, 'Race' and Ethnicity: Making Sense of the Evidence*, London: King's Fund.

Townsend, P. (1999) 'A structural plan needed to reduce inequalities of health', in D. Gordon, M. Shaw, D. Dorling and G. Davey Smith (eds) *Inequalities in Health: The Evidence*, Bristol: The Policy Press.

Tudor Hart, J. (1971) 'The inverse care law', *The Lancet*, 27 February: 405–12.

West, P. (1991) 'Rethinking the health selection explanation for health inequalities', *Social Science & Medicine* 32: 373–84.

10 The poor and the poorest*

Brian Abel-Smith and Peter Townsend

Two assumptions have governed much economic thinking in Britain since the war. The first is that we have "abolished" poverty. The second is that we are a much more equal society: that the differences between the living standards of rich and poor are much smaller than they used to be.

These assumptions are of great practical as well as theoretical importance. They form the background to much of the discussion of social and economic policy. But are they true? The findings of the survey carried out in 1950 in York by Rowntree and Lavers were encouraging.[1] They seemed to confirm expert as well as popular supposition. The absence of mass unemployment, the steady increase in the employment of married women, the post-war improvements in the social services and the increase in real wages all seemed to point unequivocally to the virtual elimination of poverty, at least as it had been understood in the nineteen-thirties.

Second, the authors of a number of studies of income distribution have found a levelling of incomes since 1938.[2] Indeed, many recent writers have concluded not only that there is less inequality of income in post-war as compared with pre-war Britain, but that the process of levelling continued during the nineteen-fifties.[3] The data produced by economists seemed merely to confirm what had been implied by the maintenance after the war of high rates of taxation, by the competition for labour in a society with relatively full employment and by the general increase in the number of persons with professional, managerial and technical skills. Both assumptions seemed to be strongly founded. [. . .]

It would of course be possible to give a long historical account of the various economic and social changes in Britain since the war. Even though there are considerable difficulties in measuring these changes in precise quantitative terms there is no doubt that the purchasing power of manual workers and of social security beneficiaries has increased substantially. There is also no doubt that during the past 20 years the number of persons holding

*This is an abridged extract from Abel-Smith, B. and Townsend, P. (1965) *The Poor and the Poorest: A New Analysis of the Ministry of Labour's Family Expenditure Surveys of 1953–54 and 1960*, Bell & Sons Ltd, pp. 9, 11–12, 57, 64–7.

the traditionally better-paid professional, managerial and skilled manual occupations has continued to increase relative to those in the semi-skilled and unskilled manual occupations – at least according to the traditional definition of 'skill'. Given the pattern of wage- and salary-levels that has existed in this country, the number and proportion of incomes in the middle ranges have tended to increase as a consequence. But beyond statements such as these it is difficult to go. The precise nature of changes in income distribution are obscure. Moreover, every generation tends to exaggerate its achievements. Those living in post-war Britain were particularly anxious to show that they had broken decisively with the past. Everyone wanted to erase the bitter memories of the thirties. By the 1950s, both major political parties had a vested interest in making the creation of the 'Welfare State' seem a greater change than it actually was. Both wanted to gain political credit for introducing it, and the Labour Party in particular wanted to gain or sustain electoral popularity because of its legislative programme of 1945–51. It was difficult for its members to tolerate criticism of its achievements or even talk about them without exaggeration. The Conservative Party had a two-fold motive – first to gain the credit for the original inspiration of the Welfare State but secondly to show that it had become unnecessarily extravagant. Middle-class anxieties about the 'burden' of taxation could be legitimated by the belief that welfare had become excessive. Certain types of information could be interpreted according to these various attitudes.

There are many features of social belief and value which deserve fuller explanation than we can attempt here. In particular the general assumption that economic and social progress has been sharper and faster than it has actually been is a sociological phenomenon of the first importance which it would be instructive to analyse. Our point is, first, that society has tended to make a rather sweeping interpretation of such evidence as there is about the reduction of poverty and the increase of equality since the war and, secondly, this evidence is a lot weaker than many social scientists have supposed. Basically, its weakness derives from conceptual rather than technical inadequacy, particularly in the sense that the measures of need and of income that have been used are more appropriate to a static than to a dynamic society.

A fresh approach is therefore called for. As a first step the income and expenditure surveys carried out by government and outside bodies, usually University departments, are likely to prove to be the most promising source for revising or obtaining information about developments in the post-war years and currently. The reports of these are tantalisingly silent on the two assumptions described at the beginning of this paper. They tell little about social conditions. They do not contain analyses of the circumstances of the poorest households in the sample in relation to conventional definitions of subsistence. Nor do they compare such households with wealthy or average households of similar or different composition. In fairness to those carrying out such surveys, they were not intended to do so. But the data could nevertheless be re-analysed in this way. [. . .]

The limited object of the work upon which this report is based was to find out from data collected in government income and expenditure surveys in two post-war years as much as possible about the levels of living and the social characteristics of the poorest section of the population in the United Kingdom. In the process we have defined and used a national assistance standard of living, have re-applied a subsistence standard adopted in an earlier study of poverty (by Rowntree and Lavers in 1950), and have given some account of the extent to which households range in income and expenditure from the average for their type. [. . .]

One conclusion that can be drawn from both surveys is that national assistance is inefficient. While it is impossible to give precise figures it is clear that substantial numbers in the population were not receiving national assistance in 1953–54 and 1960 and yet seemed, *prima facie*, to qualify for it. In the latter year, for example, there were nearly one million persons who had pensions or other state benefits and whose incomes fell below assistance rates plus rent.

This national evidence is extremely important and confirms what has been concluded from independent studies, particularly of the aged, in recent years.[4] It is given greater force by the unambiguous statement in the recent report of a Government committee of inquiry into the impact of rates on households: "We estimate that about half a million retired householders are apparently eligible for assistance but not getting it."[5]

This is not the place for a searching discussion of reforms in social security. All that we wish to point out is that there is a two-fold implication for social policy of the evidence in this report – not only that a substantial minority of the population in addition to those receiving national assistance live at or below national assistance standards, but also that a substantial minority are not receiving national assistance and yet appear to qualify for it. The legitimacy of the system of national assistance is therefore called into question.

Possibly the most novel finding is the extent of poverty among children. For over a decade it has been generally assumed that such poverty as exists is found overwhelmingly among the aged. Unfortunately it has not been possible to estimate from the data used in this study exactly how many persons over minimum pensionable age were to be found among the $7\frac{1}{2}$ million persons with low income in 1960. However, such data as we have suggest that the number may be around 3 million. There were thus more people who were not aged than were aged among the poor households of 1960. We have estimated earlier that there were about $2\frac{1}{4}$ million children in low income households in 1960. Thus quantitatively the problem of poverty among children is more than two-thirds of the size of poverty among the aged. This fact has not been given due emphasis in the policies of the political parties. It is also worth observing that there were substantially more children in poverty than adults of working age. [. . .]

Although we have tried to apply definitions and procedures which would allow the statistics for the two years to be compared, we realise that it is difficult, for technical reasons, to draw firm conclusions. Between 1953 and 1960 the Ministry of Labour surveys suggest that the number of persons living at low levels increased from 7.8 per cent to 14.2 per cent. Of the difference of 6.4 per cent we would estimate that about 1½ per cent was due to a better representation in the sample of aged persons in 1960 than in 1953 and another 0.5 or 1 per cent to a fuller representation in the sample of national assistance recipients other than the aged. Very little of the difference seems to be due to a change, relative to wages, in the definition of 'low levels of living', but part of it (about 2 per cent) seems to be due to the fact that the definition was based on income in 1960 and expenditure in 1953–54. Nonetheless, some part of the apparent increase from 7.8 to 14.2 per cent seems attributable to (*a*) the relative increase in the number of old people in the population, (*b*) a slight relative increase in the number of men in late middle age who are chronically sick, and (*c*) the relative increase in the number of families with four or more children, at a time when family allowances have increased much less than average industrial earnings and when the wages of some low-paid workers may not have increased as much as average industrial earnings. On the whole the data we have presented contradicts the commonly held view that a trend towards greater equality has accompanied the trend towards greater affluence.

In general, we regard our figures for 1960 to be the more accurate even though we believe that they understate the numbers of the population with low levels of living because of the under-representation of the aged and the sick. We may summarise our findings for that year by saying that about 5–6 per cent of the population were in low income households because wages, even when supplemented by family allowances, were insufficient to raise them above the minimum level. A further 3–4 per cent were in households receiving social insurance benefits (principally pensions) but the latter were insufficient. Many such households would probably be entitled to national assistance but for various reasons had not applied for it. A further 4–5 per cent of the population were in low income households because, under various regulations, they were not entitled to the full scale of national assistance grant or because the minimum we have taken is considerably above the *basic* national assistance scale.

Even if we take a substantially lower base line – the basic assistance scale plus rent – we find that about 2 million people (3.8 per cent of the population) were living in households with exceptionally low incomes. For about a quarter of them the problem was inadequate earnings and family allowances; for nearly half of them the problem was inadequate social insurance benefits coupled with unwillingness to apply for national assistance, and for the remainder the amount of national assistance being received was apparently inadequate.

In terms of national information we conclude from the evidence that steps should be taken by the government to ensure that regular surveys are made of the living conditions of the poorest households in our society and that reports should be published showing their sources of income and how their social characteristics compare with those of other households.

Finally, we conclude that the evidence of substantial numbers of the population living below national assistance level, and also of substantial numbers seeming to be eligible for national assistance but not receiving it, calls for a radical review of the whole social security scheme. Moreover, the fact that nearly a third of the poor were children suggests the need for a readjustment of priorities in plans for extensions and developments.

Notes

1 Rowntree, B.S., and Lavers, G.R. *Poverty and the Welfare State: A Third Social Survey of York dealing only with Economic Questions*, London, Longmans, 1951.
2 Seers, D., *The Levelling of Incomes since 1938*, Oxford, Blackwell, 1951; Cartter, A.M., *The Redistribution of Income in Post-War Britain*, New Haven, Yale University Press, 1955; Paish, F.W., "The Real Incidence of Personal Taxation", *Lloyds Bank Review*, 43, 1957, p. 1; Lydall, H.F., "The Long-Term Trend in the Size Distribution of Income", *Journal of the Royal Statistical Society*, Series A (General) *122*, Part 1, 1959, p.1.
3 "A study of the period 1938–57 reveals a continuous trend towards greater equality in the distribution of allocated personal income . . . For the future, unless there is a catastrophic slump, the trend towards equality is likely to continue, though probably not as fast as in the past twenty years." Lydall, H.F., *ibid.*, p. 34.
4 Cole, D., with Utting, J. *The Economic Circumstances of Old People*, Occasional Papers on Social Administration, No. 4, Welwyn, The Codicote Press, 1962; Townsend, P., and Wedderburn, D., *The Aged in the Welfare State*, Occasional Papers on Social Administration, No. 14, London, Bell, 1965.
5 This was a conservative estimate made after consultations with the National Assistance Board. *Report of the Committee of Inquiry into the Impact of Rates on Households* (The Allen Report), Cmnd. 2582, London, HMSO, 1965, p. 117 and pp. 221–225. The Government Social Survey carried out a special survey for the Committee in 1963 which was in all major respects identical to the family expenditure survey.

11 The Black Report*

Sir Douglas Black (Chairman)

The evidence of inequalities in health

The pattern of health inequality in contemporary Britain

Inequalities in human health take a number of distinctive forms in Britain today. In this report, most attention is given to differences in health as measured over the years between the social (or more strictly occupational) classes. These differences are highlighted in Table 1 by comparing rates of mortality among men and women in each of the Registrar General's 5 classes. Taking the two extremes as a point of comparison it can be seen that for both men and women the risk of death before retirement is two-and-a-half times as great in class V (unskilled manual workers and their wives), as it is in class I (professional men and their wives). If attention is confined to age-standardised deaths rather than all deaths of those aged 15–64 then the ratio for class V males becomes a little under twice (1.8) that of class I (OPCS, 1978, p. 37).

This great gap in the life chances of men and women at the two polar ends of the occupational spectrum is, however, not the only source of health inequality for, as Table 1 also indicates, the risk of death for men in each social class is almost twice that of their wives.

Sex differences in health

One of the most distinctive features of human health in the advanced societies is the gap in life expectancy between men and women. This phenomenon carries important implications for all spheres of social policy but especially health, since old age is a time when demand for health care is at its greatest and the dominant pattern of premature male mortality has added the exacerbating problem of isolation to the situation of elderly women who frequently survive their partners by many years. The imbalance in the ratio of males to females in old age is the cumulative product of health inequalities between the sexes during the whole lifetime. These inequalities are found in every occup-

*This is an abridged extract from Sir Douglas Black (Chairman) (1980) *Inequalities in Health – Report of a Research Working Group*, HMSO, pp. 23–8, 32–3, 35, 37–9, 91–2.

Table 1 Death rates by sex and social (occupational) class (15–64 years) (rates per 1000 pop. England and Wales, 1971)

Social (occupational) class	Males (all)	Females (married, by husbands occ.)	Ratio M/F
I (Professional)	3.98	2.15	1.85
II (Intermediate)	5.54	2.85	1.94
IIIN (Skilled non-manual)	5.80	2.76	1.96
IIIM (Skilled manual)	6.08	3.41	1.78
IV (Partly skilled)	7.96	4.27	1.87
V (Unskilled)	9.88	5.31	1.86
Ratio V/I	2.5	2.5	

Source: Occupational Mortality 1970–72. (Microfiches and 1978, p. 37).

Note: The decennial supplement of Occupational Mortality for 1970–2 provides data on the class of married and widowed women classified by (1) their present or former husband's occupation, and (2) their own occupation where this is applicable. The difference between these two measures is only significant in the case of women in class I (i.e. professional workers). When classified by their own occupation such women have somewhat lower rates of mortality from most causes than those of women allocated to class I by their husband's occupation. In this table women with husbands have been classified by their husband's occupation, women of other marital statuses are attributed to their *own* occupational class.

ational class, demonstrating that gender and class exert highly significant and different influences on the quality and duration of life in modern society.

Regional differences in health

Rates of age-specific mortality vary considerably between the regions which make up the United Kingdom. Using mortality as an indicator of health, the healthiest part of Britain appears to be in the southern belt (below a line drawn across the country from the Wash to the Bristol Channel). This part of the country has not always exhibited the low rates of mortality that are found there today. In the middle of the nineteenth century, the South East of England recorded comparatively high rates of death, while other regions like Wales and the far North had a rather healthier profile. The fluctuation in the distribution of mortality over the years suggests that social (including industrial and occupational) as much as "natural" factors must be at work in creating the pattern of regional health inequalities. Table 2 depicts regional variation in mortality standardised for age and for both age and occupational class. Once again it is clear that these variables exert, at least statistically, an independent influence on human health.

Race, ethnicity and health

One of the most important dimensions of inequality in contemporary Britain is race. Immigrants to this country from the so-called New Commonwealth, whose ethnic identity is clearly visible in the colour of their skin, are known to

Table 2 Regional variations in mortality

Standard region	SMR: standardised for	
	Age	Age and class
Northern, Yorkshire and Humberside	113	113
North West	106	105
East Midlands	116	116
West Midlands	96	94
East Anglia	105	104
South East	90	90
South West	93	93
Wales I	114	117
Wales II	110	113
England and Wales	100	100

Source: Occupational Mortality 1970–72, p. 180.

experience greater difficulty in finding work and adequate housing (Smith, 1976). Given, for example, these social and economic disabilities it is to be expected that they might also record rather higher than average rates of mortality and morbidity.

This hypothesis is difficult to test from official statistics, since "race" has rarely been assessed in official censuses and surveys. Moreover, it is far from clear what indicator should be utilized in any such assessment (e.g. skin-colour, place of birth, nationality): that most significant may indeed depend upon the precise issue of interest.

The pattern of social and economic disadvantage experienced by black Britons is connected with occupational class and is reflected in the working of the labour market. But other factors may also be important and amongst adult males at least, the variables of occupational class and race do not compound one another in a linear fashion when place of birth is used as a means of measuring race. As Table 3 indicates, the age standardised mortality ratios of immigrant males compare favourably with their British born equivalents in occupational classes IV and V, but less so higher up in the scale in classes I and II. The interpretation of these ratios is made difficult at the higher end of the occupational scale because they are based on small numbers.

Table 3 Mortality by country of birth and occupational class (SMR) (Males 15–64)

Country of birth	I	II	IIIN	IIIM	IV	V	All
India and Pakistan	122	127	114	105	93	73	98
West Indies	267	163	135	87	71	75	84
Europe (including UK & Eire)	121	109	98	83	81	82	89
UK & Eire (including England and Wales)	118	112	111	118	115	110	114
England and Wales	97	99	99	99	99	100	100
All birth places	100	100	100	100	100	100	100

Source: Occupational Mortality, 1970–72, pp. 186–187.

In the poorer occupational classes, where the SMR is based on larger numbers of deaths, men born in India, Pakistan or the West Indies seem to live longer than their British born counterparts. It should be remembered, however, that the percentage of workers in class V among the British born is less than 7 while the equivalent percentage of those born in, for example, India and Pakistan is 16. In addition, of course, the average British born male classified as an unskilled manual worker is likely to be older than his foreign born counterpart and is more likely to have acquired this low occupational status after a process of downward social mobility associated with failing health.

This rather favourable comparison between immigrant and British born males may also reflect the underlying tendency for migrants to select themselves on the grounds of health and fitness. Men and women prepared to cross oceans and continents in order to seek new occupational opportunities or a new way of life do not represent a random cross-section of humanity. A better comparison for exploring health inequality would ideally involve second or third generation immigrants, but these are the very groups that are difficult to trace for statistical purposes. What little evidence that has been accumulated however does suggest that the children of immigrants do suffer from certain specific health disabilities related to cultural factors such as diet or to their lack of natural immunity to certain infectious diseases (Thomas, 1968; Oppé, 1967; Gans, 1966). Studies based on small samples of immigrant children have pointed to the possibility of higher than average morbidity associated with material deprivation but the evidence is scarce and somewhat inconclusive and needs to be augmented by further research (Hood *et al.*, 1970).

Social class and health

Social class is a further concept by means of which inequalities in industrial society may be examined. It reflects income, property, occupation and education, and much else. The data presented in the remainder of this chapter employ occupation as a means of approximating social class [. . .].

Mortality

Contemporary trends in occupational mortality have been extensively reviewed in the most recent decennial supplement of occupational mortality (OPCS, 1978). A summary of some of the most relevant findings will be presented here.

Class differences in mortality are a constant feature of the entire human lifetime. They are found at birth, during the first year of life, in childhood, adolescence and in adult life. In general they are more marked at the start of life and in early adulthood. Average life expectancy provides a useful summary of the cumulative impact of these advantages and disadvantages throughout life. A child born to professional parents, if he or she is not socially mobile, can expect to spend over 5 years more as a living person than a child born to an unskilled manual household. [. . .]

At birth and during the first month of life the risk of death in class V (unskilled manual workers) is double the risk in class I (professional workers). When the fortunes of babies born to skilled manual fathers (class IIIM) are compared with those who enter the world as the offspring of professional workers (class I) the risk of mortality is one and a half times as great. From the end of the first month to the end of the first year, class differentials in infant mortality reach a peak of disadvantage. For the death of every one male infant in class I, we can expect almost 2 deaths in class IIIM and 4 deaths in class V. [. . .]

Between the ages of one and fourteen, the risk of mortality continues to be closely correlated with class. Among boys the ratio of mortality in V as compared with I is of the order of 2:1, among the girls it varies between 1.5:−1 to 1.9:1. Once again the cause of this difference can be traced to environmental origins. The most steep gradients in childhood are found for accidents (33 per cent of total causes). For deaths caused by fire, falls and drowning the risk for boys in class V is 10 times the risk for their peers in class I. The corresponding ratio for deaths caused to youthful pedestrians by motor vehicles is more than 7:1. The other major causes of death showing step class gradients in childhood are infective and parasitic disease (5 per cent of the total) and pneumonia (8 per cent of the total). For most other causes, there is less clear evidence of class disadvantage.

Class differences in mortality for all adults aged 15–64 are somewhat less marked than in childhood, but this conceals a large difference for those in their 20s and 30s, and a small difference for those approaching pension age, i.e. class disadvantage becomes less extreme as men and women grow older and the frequency of death increases. The risk of death in class V is between one and a half to two times the risk in class I for adult males and females. [. . .]

In adult life, class differences in mortality are found for many different causes. As in childhood the rate of accidental death and infectious disease forms a steep gradient especially among men; moreover an extraordinary variety of causes of deaths such as cancer, heart and respiratory disease, also differentiate between the classes. [. . .]

Conclusion

Our review of trends in inequalities of health has produced some disturbing conclusions.

As explained earlier in the chapter, trends are not easy to trace, either because of inconsistencies in the categorisation of data or changes in occupational classification. Our conclusions make allowance for these problems. We have also had the opportunity of comparing trends in infant mortality with trends in mortality of people at later ages. Analyses in the literature have tended to concentrate attention either on infant mortality or mortality of males of economically active age rather than on the population of both sexes of different age.

Perhaps the most important general finding in the chapter is the lack of improvement, and indeed in some respects deterioration, of the health experience not merely of occupational class V but also class IV in health, relative to occupational class I, as judged by mortality indicators, during the 1960s and early 1970s. The more specific conclusions, underlying this finding, are as follows. (These conclusions, apply to England and Wales. Scottish experience has been rather similar, though certain differences are noted in the text.)

i   Mortality rates of males are higher at every age than of females and in recent decades the difference between the sexes has become relatively greater.

ii   For men of economically active age there was greater inequality of mortality between occupational classes I and V both in 1970–72 and 1959–63 than in 1949–53.

iii   For economically active men the mortality rates of occupational class III and combined classes IV and V for age-groups over 35 either deteriorated or showed little or no improvement between 1959–63 and 1970–72. Relative to the mortality rates of occupational classes I and II they worsened.

iv   For women aged 15–64 the standardised mortality ratios of combined classes IV and V deteriorated. For married and single women in class IV (the most numerous class) they deteriorated at all ages.

v   Although deaths per thousand live births in England and Wales have diminished among all classes the relative excess in combined classes IV and V over I and II increased between 1959–63 and 1970–72.

vi   During a period of less than a decade maternal mortality fell by more than a third. Although that of class I fell less sharply than other classes inequality between the more numerous class II and classes IV and V remained about the same.

vii   Among children between 1 and 4 years of age, there has been a small reduction in the class differential (especially for girls), for children aged 5 to 9 little or no change, but for children aged 10 to 14 an increase in the differential. For boys aged 1–14, mortality ratios for classes IV and V in 1970–72 were *both* higher than for classes I and II for 23 of 38 causes of death, compared with only one cause (asthma) where the ratios were lower. For girls the corresponding figures were 22 and 0 respectively. There is evidence that as rates of child death from a specific condition decline to very low levels class gradients do disappear. The gradual elimination of death from rheumatic heart disease over the post war period provides evidence of this (Morris, 1959).

References

Gans, B., "Health Problems and the Immigrant Child", in CIBA Foundation, *Immigration: Medical and Social Aspects*, 1966.

Hood, C., Oppé, T.E., Pless, I.B. and Apte, E., *West Indian Immigrants: A Study of One-year olds in Paddington*, Institute of Race Relations, 1970.

Morris, J.N., "Health and Social Class" *The Lancet* February 7th, 1959.

OPCS, *Occupational Mortality 1970–72, Decennial Supplement*, London, HMSO, 1978.

Oppé, T.E., "The Health of West Indian Children", *Proc. Roy. Soc. Med.*, 57, 1967, pp. 321–323.

Smith, D., *The Facts of Racial Disadvantage: A National Survey*, London, PEP, 1976.

Thomas, H.E., "Tuberculosis in Immigrants", *Proc. Roy. Soc. Med.*, 61, 1968.

12 Widening inequality of health in northern England, 1981–91*

Peter Phillimore, Alastair Beattie and Peter Townsend

Introduction

Several studies have indicated widening social class differences in mortality in Britain in the 1970s,[1-8] indeed, a widening gap can be traced back to the 1950s.[9] Given this long trend towards widening inequality in health, it would be surprising if differences in mortality were found to narrow in the 1980s, and increasing disparities in mortality through the 1980s have already been reported for Glasgow.[10] The decade has been one of profound social and economic change, with two major recessions, a widening of income differentials,[11] and a reduction of the real income of the poorest 10% of households in the population.[12] Nevertheless, changes in mortality among different sections of the population need careful identification. In this paper we examine relative and absolute changes in mortality (all causes) in people aged under 75 between 1981 and 1991 in the area administered by Northern Regional Health Authority (the five counties of Cleveland, Cumbria, Durham, Northumberland, and Tyne and Wear). This builds on our earlier study of inequalities in health in this region of three million people.[1,2]

Methods

Socioeconomic and population data were drawn from the 1981 and 1991 censuses and mortality data (1981–91) were taken from death records of the Office of Population Censuses and Surveys for the 678 wards used in our earlier study.[1,2] The index of deprivation created previously was reconstructed with data from the 1991 census. This index was constructed by means of z scores, combining four variables selected to reflect distinctive aspects of material wellbeing – unemployment, car ownership, non-owner occupation, and household overcrowding. Any method of combining several variables with different distributions into a single index will have drawbacks,[13] but the z score is widely used and at ward level gives similar results to other methods.[14]

*This article was first published in the *British Medical Journal*, vol. 308, pp. 1125–8, 1994.

The populations in the 1981 census provided denominators for deaths in 1981–4, as did the populations in the 1991 census for deaths in 1988–91. The mean of the 1981 and 1991 populations was used as a denominator for deaths occurring in 1985–7. This enabled us to review mortality throughout the decade. Standardised mortality ratios were calculated for each ward over 11 years, but deaths were usually grouped into successive periods of three years. Absolute changes were examined by recalculating mortality ratios for 1989–91, standardising to rates in England and Wales in 1981–3. The ratio of the standardised mortality ratios for 1989–91 and 1981–3 was then calculated.[15] To identify whether inequalities in mortality had widened, wards were grouped into fifths according to the levels of deprivation reflected in the summary z score for 1981 or 1991 with additional information about the highest and lowest tenths.

Population denominators refer to residents in households. Accordingly, deaths of people living in institutions were removed from the analysis. With regard to the accuracy of 1991 census population counts, underenumeration appears to have been less in the Northern region than nationally: imputed residents (reflecting the gap between census counts and estimates of the real population) accounted for 0.89% of the population in households in the Northern region, compared with 1.64% in England and Wales.[16] Both nationally and in the Northern region underenumeration was most pronounced among young adults, particularly men in their twenties.[17] Because underenumeration was understood to be largely a consequence of homelessness and avoidance of poll tax it might be expected to be more pronounced in deprived than affluent populations. To check the social distribution of this deficit, we examined population changes in each five year age band in the most deprived fifth of wards, comparing the ratio of men to women in each age band between 1981 and 1991 as a guide to anomalies in the 1991 population structure of these poor wards. This exercise confirmed an apparent deficit of men in the 20–34 age group, in which numbers of men should have been 15.3% higher if trends had mirrored the female population. However, because deaths are much more numerous in the 35–44 age group than in the younger age group, there is only a small effect on mortality in the 15–44 age range as a whole. Comparing changes in the proportions of expected deaths for men and women aged 15–44 for 1981–3 and for 1989–91 shows that expected deaths in men should be just 2.7% higher than the value calculated with published population data.

Results

Table 1 shows socioeconomic data for 1981 and 1991. The high levels of unemployment in the poorest wards at both censuses persisted throughout the decade and peaked in 1986. Of the four indicators composing the deprivation index, only overcrowding showed a general decline. Overall, there was little change in the relative position of wards between 1981 and 1991. A

Table 1 Distribution of indicators of deprivation in 678 electoral wards in Northern region in 1981 and 1991. Values are percentages unless stated otherwise

Grouping of wards by deprivation (No. of wards)*	People unemployed	Households with no car	Households not owner occupied	Households overcrowded	Total population (No)
1981					
Most deprived tenth (68)	23.5	70.4	82.9	7.1	474,037
Most deprived fifth (136)	21.0	65.6	76.3	6.2	900,501
Second fifth (136)	14.1	52.8	59.6	4.0	683,348
Third fifth (134)	11.1	46.1	47.3	2.9	587,867
Fourth fifth (136)	8.1	33.8	34.0	2.0	447,234
Least deprived fifth (136)	6.0	21.4	18.8	1.2	415,024
Least deprived tenth (68)	5.4	19.4	14.8	0.9	232,894
1991					
Most deprived tenth (68)	24.0	66.8	67.9	3.0	427,491
Most deprived fifth (136)	20.6	61.5	61.0	2.6	799,860
Second fifth (136)	12.7	47.6	43.8	1.6	727,398
Third fifth (134)	9.1	37.7	33.7	1.2	566,092
Fourth fifth (136)	6.6	27.7	23.0	0.8	487,678
Least deprived fifth (136)	4.6	16.0	13.3	0.5	405,328
Least deprived tenth (68)	4.1	13.0	11.0	0.4	195,933

*Wards ranked on basis of 1981 deprivation index for 1981 data and 1991 deprivation index for 1991 data.

Spearman rank correlation coefficient of 0.96 between deprivation z scores for the two periods confirmed this similarity. Only 19 of the 136 wards making up the region's poorest fifth in 1981 were outside this fifth in 1991. Such stability was reflected across the socioeconomic spectrum.

Table 2 shows the mortality data for people aged under 65, which suggest that inequalities in mortality had widened over the decade. A clear worsening of mortality relative to the national level in the poorest fifth of wards was accompanied by little relative change in the second and middle fifths and an improvement in the most affluent 40% of wards. Table 3 shows the wards with highest and lowest mortality in the region, illustrating how pronounced localised disparities were during 1981–91. At this level of analysis, mortality in the most favoured areas was one quarter of the rate found in the worst affected localities.

Table 4 summarises the mortality of specific age groups during 1981–91 in the most deprived fifth and most affluent fifth of wards. Ward groupings are based solely on the 1981 deprivation ranking so that the same localities were compared over time. Since the deprived wards were located predominantly in the major urban centres, where wards cover larger populations than in small towns and rural areas, there was a large difference in the sizes of the populations compared. In 1991 the poorest fifth of wards included 28% of the region's population, while the richest fifth included 15% of the total. In each

Table 2 Association between mortality ratios and deprivation in people aged under 65 in electoral wards in Northern region during 1981–3 and 1989–91

Grouping of wards by deprivation*	1981–3		1989–91	
	Mortality ratio†	No. of deaths	Mortality ratio†	No. of deaths
Most deprived tenth	145	5,601	158	4,356
Most deprived fifth	136	10,081	150	7,807
Second fifth	120	6,642	121	5,864
Third fifth	109	5,063	111	4,134
Fourth fifth	100	3,610	92	3,078
Least deprived fifth	87	2,746	84	2,346
Least deprived tenth	84	1,490	81	1,123
Ratio of most deprived tenth to least deprived	1.73		1.95	

*Groupings for 1981–3 based on 1981 deprivation rank and for 1989–91 on 1991 deprivation rank.
† 1981–3 standardised to national (England Wales) mortality in 1981–3; 1989–91 standardised to national mortality in 1989–91.

Table 3 Level of deprivation in the six electoral wards in Northern region with highest mortality in 1981–91 and the six with lowest mortality

Ward and local authority	Mortality ratio (95% confidence interval)*	Deprivation rank†	
		1981	1991
Highest mortality			
St Hilda's (Middlesbrough)	217 (191 to 245)	10	17
West City (Newcastle)	203 (184 to 223)	3	1
Portrack and Tilery (Stockton)	194 (173 to 217)	48	29
Grangetown (Langbaurgh)	187 (161 to 215)	14	6
Southfield (Middlesbrough)	186 (160 to 213)	44	34
Deneside (Easington)	183 (160 to 206)	28	12
Lowest mortality			
Gosforth (Copeland)	57 (36 to 82)	574	639
Redesdale (Tynedale)	55 (29 to 88)	499	519
Crosby Ravensworth (Eden)	52 (30 to 80)	625	535
Hummersknott (Darlington)	51 (39 to 65)	672	664
Wylam (Tynedale)	51 (34 to 71)	624	625
Whalton (Castle Morpeth)	46 (23 to 76)	520	522

*Standardised to national (England and Wales 1981–91) mortality of 100.
† Range from 1 (most deprived) to 678 (least deprived).

age range the gap between the most deprived and the most affluent areas seemed to have widened. This was not invariably because of improvements in standardised mortality ratios in the most affluent wards: only in the 15–44 age range was a substantial improvement evident. In general the widening gap was mainly due to standardised mortality ratios rising in the poorest wards. The position of the populations of the poorest wards worsened over the decade in

Table 4 Trends in age specific mortality in most deprived and least deprived fifths of electoral wards in Northern region. Values are standardised mortality ratios* (numbers of people)

	Age group of most deprived fifth of wards				
	0–14	15–44	45–54	55–64	65–74
1981–3	116 (620)	117 (1,116)	130 (2,041)	145 (6,304)	123 (9,562)
1983–5	117 (580)	119 (1,085)	135 (1,892)	149 (6,206)	122 (9,256)
1985–7	119 (588)	120 (1,072)	145 (1,778)	151 (5,789)	127 (9,441)
1987–9	114 (551)	128 (1,141)	152 (1,624)	153 (5,302)	130 (9,474)
1989–91	130 (566)	128 (1,144)	162 (1,575)	151 (4,745)	133 (9,397)
	Age group of least deprived fifth of wards				
	0–14	15–44	45–54	55–64	65–74
1981–3	80 (195)	86 (428)	79 (574)	92 (1,549)	94 (3,178)
1983–5	77 (170)	84 (406)	81 (560)	96 (1,626)	90 (3,042)
1985–7	70 (145)	87 (427)	79 (546)	88 (1,531)	87 (2,962)
1987–9	71 (135)	79 (400)	78 (535)	85 (1,460)	87 (2,995)
1989–91	79 (131)	77 (390)	83 (549)	87 (1,433)	88 (2,981)

*Standardised to national (England and Wales) mortality of 100 in each three year period. Local population denominators: 1981 census for deaths in 1981–4: 1986 population (derived from 1981 and 1991 censuses) for deaths in 1985–7; and 1991 census for deaths in 1988–91. Deprivation defined on basis of 1981 census.

all age categories, but this was most pronounced in the 45–54 age range. A widening of the differential among those aged 65–74 also supports evidence of inequalities persisting beyond retirement.[18]

The possibility that the widening gap among younger adults might in part be attributable to underenumeration at the 1991 census disproportionately affecting the poorest wards can be discounted. When the standardised mortality ratio for the 15–44 age range in 1989–91 in the poorest wards shown in table 4 was adjusted to take account of the deficit of young men it fell only from 128 to 127. Moreover, the actual number of deaths in men aged 15–44 in the poorest fifth of wards increased from 726 in 1981–3 to 772 in 1989–91. This increase in a population that, even after adjustment for underenumeration, had fallen emphasises that the evidence for some widening of inequality should be taken as seriously in this age category as in others.

Table 5 shows standardised mortality ratios for 1981–3 and 1989–91, both standardised to national data for 1981–3, to examine absolute changes in the most and least deprived fifths of wards. In the affluent areas all age categories exhibit a distinct improvement, with significant reductions (P<0.05) in each category except for one (women aged 15–44). In the poor areas the picture is uneven. There were significant reductions (P<0.05) among children and men aged 55–64 and 65–74, although improvements were less than in the affluent wards. In other age categories improvements were small or non-existent. Among men aged 45–54 mortality was unchanged, while among women aged 65–74 mortality slightly increased. The possible importance of this deterior-

Table 5 Absolute changes in mortality between 1981–3 and 1989–91 in most deprived and least deprived* fifths of electoral wards in Northern region

| Age group | Mortality ratios† for most deprived wards | | % change (95% confidence interval) |
	1981–3 (total population 900,501)	1989–91 (total population 829,453)	
			Males and females
0–64	136	124	−9 (−12 to −7)
0–14	116	99	−15 (−24 to −5)
			Males
0–64	137	123	−10 (−13 to −7)
15–44	117	131	12 (1 to 24)
45–54	137	137	−1 (−8 to 8)
55–64	144	120	−17 (−21 to −13)
65–74	124	113	−9 (−13 to −6)
			Females
0–64	136	125	−8 (−12 to −3)
15–44	117	106	−9 (−21 to 5)
45–54	127	119	−6 (−16 to 4)
55–64	146	138	−5 (−11 to 1)
65–74	123	127	3 (−1 to 8)

| Age group | Mortality ratios† for least deprived wards | | % change (95% confidence interval) |
	1981–3 (total population 415,024)	1989–92 (total population 433,517)	
			Males and females
0–64	87	70	−20 (−24 to −15)
0–14	80	60	−25 (−40 to −7)
			Males
0–64	85	66	−22 (−27 to −17)
15–44	84	69	−18 (−31 to −2)
45–54	79	66	−16 (−28 to −2)
55–64	90	67	−25 (−31 to −17)
65–74	94	75	−20 (−25 to −15)
			Females
0–64	91	76	−16 (−23 to −8)
15–44	90	76	−16 (−33 to 4)
45–54	84	67	−20 (−34 to −4)
55–64	95	81	−15 (−24 to −4)
65–74	95	82	−14 (−20 to −7)

*Deprivation defined on basis of 1981 census.
† Standardised to national (England and Wales 1981–3) mortality of 100.

ation should not be underestimated because a similar pattern also occurred in the second most deprived fifth of wards. Among men aged 15–44 there was a larger increase in mortality. When the male population was adjusted to match changes in the female population this increase reduced but only from 12% (95% confidence interval 1% to 24%) to 9% (−2% to 20%). These patterns in the more deprived areas were apparent in all parts of the Northern region, but the Teesside conurbation contributed disproportionately to the trend in mortality among men aged under 55.

These results underline how closely health and wealth are related. Moreover, the statistical association between deprivation and mortality at ward level is greatly strengthened by combining data for an extended period. A Spearman rank correlation coefficient, weighted by the inverse of the variance around the mortality estimates, for the association between standardised mortality ratio for people aged under 65 during 1981–91 and deprivation rank (in both 1981 and 1991) was 0.85. This contrasts with a similar coefficient of 0.69 for mortality in 1981–83 and deprivation in 1981,[1,2] when small numbers of deaths in rural wards with low populations weakened the underlying strength of the relationship over a short period.[19]

Discussion

In a region that includes some of the poorest areas in Britain mortality differentials have continued to widen through the 1980s. Not only has mortality worsened in relative terms at all ages up to 75 in the poorest fifth of wards, but mortality in absolute terms has scarcely changed for several age categories over the decade relative to 1981–3 and has worsened in two categories. This runs counter to the general secular decline in death rates.[20] Most striking is evidence of the poorest areas increasingly coming adrift from the experience of the rest of the population. But even without the experience of the most deprived fifth of wards there has been no narrowing of inequality in mortality across the remainder of the population, countering suggestions that continuing health inequalities largely reflect the high mortality of a small and shrinking section of the population.[21-23] Mortality experience in poor areas continues to lag far behind average national experience, particularly in middle age. In the poorest 10% of wards mortality in 1989–91 among men aged 45–54 and women aged 55–64 was equivalent to national (England and Wales) levels of mortality last experienced in the late 1940s, while among women aged 45–54 and men aged 55–64 the equivalent national rates occurred in the early 1950s.[24]

The data on mortality among men aged 15–44 contribute to the understanding of a national phenomenon. Since 1985 deaths rates among 15–44 year olds have risen nationally, especially in men.[25] Dunnell has shown that this rise may be explained by an increasing proportion of 40–44 year olds within this wide age range, but she also noted that after adjustment for the skewed distribution of this population death rates have remained level, whereas mortality at other ages has continued to fall.[26] She suggested that AIDS might be the main contributor to the remaining anomaly among 15–44 year old men. Although we have not analysed deaths by cause, our evidence casts doubt on this assumption. In the Northern region the pattern of change among 15–44 year olds was highly differentiated. While mortality rose in the poorest fifth of wards, it changed little in the next two fifths, fell modestly in the fourth (down

- Several studies reported widening differences in mortality among social classes in Britain in the 1970s
- In this study the association between deprivation and mortality during the 1980s was studied in electoral wards in the Northern region of England
- During 1981–91 inequalities in mortality widened in men and women of all age categories under 75 years, primarily because of the situation in poorest areas worsening relative to the rest of the population
- In absolute terms mortality fell substantially in all age categories in the most affluent wards, while in some age categories in the poorest wards it actually increased, especially in men aged 15–44
- These results re-emphasise the link between public health and material conditions rather than individual behaviour

Figure 1 Public health implications.

7%), and fell most in the richest fifth of wards. This suggests that structural factors such as deregulation at work and unemployment are probably at least as influential as the developing impact of HIV and AIDS on national changes in mortality among men aged 15–44.

The most widely distributed adverse pattern was the slight increase in mortality among women aged 65–74 in the poorest 40% of wards. It is not clear why mortality should have risen in this age group but fallen among 55–64 year olds. However, much of the fall in the overall number of deaths in those aged under 65 in the most deprived wards is attributable to absolute improvements in mortality in the 55–64 range, particularly among men, which tends to obscure more disturbing trends at other ages.

A recent review of literature on health inequalities since the Black report noted with dismay a current preoccupation with behavioural explanations for health differentials,[3,6] and our evidence supports those studies which challenge this preoccupation with behaviour.[27–30] If health differentials reflected behavioural choices by individuals then worsening health would be an indication of increasingly unwise personal behaviour. Yet if historical improvements in health throughout the population are generally attributed to rising living standards and improving material conditions, so worsening health among some groups and widening differentials must be related primarily to changes in the same factors.

In this context the indicators in table 1 reveal an incomplete picture of social change and growing inequality. Thus, households with two cars (highly correlated with income) increased considerably over the decade in affluent groups, while long term unemployment featured disproportionately among those unemployed in the poorest areas. There are other limitations in relying exclusively on the census for the interpretation of trends in health. Its emphasis on individuals and households takes no account of differences between areas in the economic infrastructure of services and aspects of the physical environment such as air and water quality. National data on income distribution offer one compensating source, however, as Wilkinson has shown.[4,31,32] Official statistics reveal widening income differentials in Britain during the 1980s, particularly since 1985, on a range of indicators (that is, gross, post-tax, and disposable incomes).[11,33] Over the same period there has been an enormous growth in the population living on less than half of average income, with the poorest 10% of households suffering a fall in real income;[12] this is a trend fuelled not only by the continuation of high levels of unemployment but also by changes in the tax and state benefit systems.[34] The area administered by Northern Regional Health Authority has the highest proportion of households in low income categories in England and Wales.[35] How far the effects on health of these structural changes in society have yet emerged in mortality remains open to question. This study raises the possibility that some of these effects on ill health may just be starting to appear.

We thank Northern Regional Health Authority for its support, which made this study possible, and thank in particular Angus McNay, David Morris, and Valerie Lockie for their help. We also thank Bruce Charlton, Chris Foy, David Gordon, Michael Hill, Richard Wilkinson, and two anonymous referees for the BMJ for their helpful comments and advice.

References

1 Townsend P, Phillimore P, Beattie A. *Health and deprivation: inequality and the north.* London: Routledge, 1988.

2 Townsend P, Phillimore P, Beattie A. *Inequalities in health in the Northern region: an interim report.* Newcastle upon Tyne: Northern Regional Health Authority and Bristol University, 1986.

3 Davey Smith G, Bartley M, Blane D. The Black report on socioeconomic inequalities in health 10 years on. *BMJ* 1990;**301**:373–7.

4 Wilkinson R. Class mortality differentials, income distribution and trends in poverty 1921–1981. *Journal of Social Policy* 1989;**18**:307–35.

5 Marmot M, McDowall M. Mortality decline and widening social inequalities. *Lancet* 1986;ii:274–6.

6 Townsend P, Davidson N, Whitehead M. *Inequalities in health: the Black report and the health divide.* Harmondsworth: Penguin, 1988.

7 Goldblatt P. Mortality by social class, 1971–85. *Population Trends* 1989;**56**:6–15.

8 Blane D, Davey Smith G, Bartley M. Social class differences in years of potential life lost: size, trends, and principal causes. *BMJ* 1990;**301**:429–32.

9 Pamuk E. Social class inequality in mortality from 1921 to 1972 in England and Wales. *Population Studies* 1985;**39**:17–31.

10 Forwell G. *Glasgow's health: old problems – new opportunities. A report by the director of public health.* Glasgow: Department of Public Health, 1993.

11 Central Statistical Office. Trends in income distribution, 1977–1990. *Economic Trends* 1993;**471**:187.

12 Department of Social Security. *Households below average income 1979–1990/91.* London: HMSO, 1993.

13 Thunhurst C. The analysis of small area statistics and planning for health. *Statistician* 1985;**34**:93–106.

14 Morphet C. The interpretation of small area census data. *Area* 1992;**24**:63–72.

15 Morris JA, Gardner MJ. Calculating confidence intervals for relative risks (odds ratios) and standardised ratios and rates. *BMJ* 1988;**296**:1313–6.

16 Office of Population Censuses and Surveys. *1991 census report for Great Britain.* Parts 1 and 2. London: HMSO, 1993.

17 Population Statistics Division, Office of Population Censuses and Surveys. How complete was the 1991 census? *Population Trends* 1993;**71**:22–5.

18 Fox A, Goldblatt P, Jones D. Social class mortality differentials: artefact, selection or life circumstances? *J Epidemiol Community Health* 1985;**39**:1–8.

19 Phillimore P, Reading R. A rural advantage? Urban-rural health differences in northern England. *J Public Health Med* 1992;**14**:290–9.

20 Murray C, Chen L. In search of a contemporary theory for understanding mortality change. *Soc Sci Med* 1993;**36**:143–55.

21 Strong P. Black on class and mortality: theory, method and history. *J Public Health Med* 1990;**12**:168–80.

22 Illsley R. Occupational class, selection and the production of inequalities in health. *Quarterly Journal of Social Affairs* 1986;**2**:151–65.

23 Illsley R. Occupational class, selection and inequalities in health: a rejoinder to Richard Wilkinson's reply. *Quarterly Journal of Social Affairs* 1987;**3**:213–23.

24 Registrar General. *Statistical review of England and Wales, part 1, medical.* London: HMSO, 1950–9. (Annual.)

25 Department of Health. *On the state of the public health. Annual report of the chief medical officer of the Department of Health for the year 1990.* London: HMSO, 1990.

26 Dunnell K. Deaths among 15–44 year olds. *Population Trends* 1991;**64**:38–43.

27 Blaxter M. *Health and lifestyles.* London: Tavistock, 1990.

28 Graham H. *Women, health and the family.* Brighton: Wheatsheaf, 1984.

29 Hart N. The social and economic environment and human health. In: Holland W, Detels R, Knox G, eds. *Oxford textbook of public health.* Vol I. 2nd ed. Oxford: Oxford University Press, 1991:151–80.

30 Sterling T. Does smoking kill workers or does working kill smokers? Or the relationship between smoking, occupation and respiratory disease. *Int J Health Serv* 1978;**8**:437–52.

31 Wilkinson R. Income distribution and mortality: a "natural" experiment. *Sociology of Health and Illness* 1990;**12**:391–412.

32 Wilkinson R. The impact of income inequality on life expectancy. In: Platt S, Thomas H, Scott S, Williams G, eds. *Locating health: sociological and historical explorations.* Aldershot: Avebury, 1993;7–28.

33 Atkinson A. *What is happening to the distribution of income in the United Kingdom?* London: STICERD, London School of Economics, 1993.

34 Oppenheim C. *Poverty: the facts.* London: Child Poverty Action Group, 1992.

35 Central Statistical Office. *Regional trends 28.* London HMSO, 1993:101.

13 What makes women sick*

Lesley Doyal

A picture of health?

All women whose physical or mental health is damaged will therefore be harmed in broadly similar ways, and morbidity and mortality rates can give us a preliminary indication of the global distribution of this harm. Of course such statistics can provide only a partial picture since they are not measuring the subjective or experiential aspects of illness. Moreover they offer a negative view of sickness and death rather than a positive picture of well-being. However they do represent important points of reference between societies and social groups as well as offering clues to structural factors underlying any perceived inequalities.

Inequalities in mortality

In most of the developed countries women can now expect to survive for about 75 years (United Nations, 1991, p. 55). However this average conceals significant variations in life expectancy between women in different social groups. In Britain women married to men in semi-skilled or unskilled jobs are about 70 per cent more likely to die prematurely than those whose husbands are professionals (OPCS, 1986). Similar social divisions are apparent in the United States, where black women now have a life expectancy of 73.5 years compared with 79.2 for white women while their risk of dying in pregnancy or childbirth is three and a half times greater (US National Institutes of Health, 1992, pp. 8, 13). In most underdeveloped countries the social inequalities in health are even more dramatic.

There are also major differences in mortality rates between rich and poor nations. In Latin America and the Caribbean average life expectancy is lower than in developed countries but still relatively high at around 70. In Asia and the Pacific it is 64 and in Africa as low as 54 (UN, 1991, p. 55). The lowest rates recorded for individual countries are in Afghanistan, East Timor,

*This is an extract from Doyal, L. (1995) *What Makes Women Sick: Gender and the Political Economy of Health*, Macmillan Press, pp. 10–15.

Ethiopia and Sierra Leone, where women can expect to live for only about 43 years (ibid.) These inequalities are at their most extreme in deaths related to childbearing. In developed countries mortality of this kind is rare, with less than five deaths for every 100 000 live births. In South Asian countries, on the other hand, the rate is more than 650 deaths per 100 000 with the African average a close second at around 600 deaths (UN, 1991, p. 56).

Though these figures are extremely dramatic they do not show the true extent of the inequalities in reproductive hazards facing women in different parts of the world. The maternal mortality rate reflects the risk a woman runs in each pregnancy. However we also need to examine fertility rates to assess the lifetime risk to an individual woman of dying of pregnancy-related causes. Recent estimates suggest that for a woman in Africa this risk is 1 in 23 compared with only 1 in 10 000 in developed countries (Rooney, 1992). Pregnancy causes almost no deaths among women of reproductive age in developed countries but between a quarter and a third of deaths elsewhere (Fortney *et al.*, 1986). Reproductive deaths are therefore an important indicator both of the different health hazards facing men and women and also of the heterogeneity of women's own experiences.

Turning from mortality to morbidity statistics – from death to disease – we are immediately faced with what appears to be a paradox. Around the world, women usually live longer than men in the same socio-economic circumstances. In most of the developed countries the gap between male and female life expectancy is about 6.5 years (UN, 1991, p. 55). In Latin America and the Caribbean it is 5.0 years, in Africa 3.5 years and in Asia and the Pacific, 3.0 years (ibid.). Only in a few countries in Asia do women have a lower life expectancy than men. Yet despite their generally greater longevity, women in most communities report more illness and distress. This pattern of excess female morbidity is reasonably well documented in the developed countries and we examine that evidence first. The more limited information on women in third world countries will be considered later.

Sickness and affluence

A number of studies in the United Kingdom have found that women's own assessment of their health is consistently worse than that of men (Blaxter, 1990; Whitehead, 1988). Similar findings have emerged from studies in the United States (Rodin and Ickovics, 1990; Verbrugge, 1986). US women are 25 per cent more likely than men to report that their activities are restricted by health problems and they are bedridden for 35 per cent more days than men because of acute conditions (US National Institutes of Health, 1992, p. 9). In community surveys throughout the developed world, women report about twice as much anxiety and depression as men (Paykel, 1991; Weissman and Klerman, 1977).

Women also use most medical services more often. This fact cannot be taken as a straightforward indicator of the relative well-being of the two sexes since admitting illness may well be more acceptable for women than for men. However it does highlight certain important features of women's health status. The most immediate reason for their greater use of medical care is longevity. Deteriorating health and increasing disability are a frequent, though not inevitable accompaniment of the ageing process and women make up a large proportion of the elderly in the population – especially the 'old old' (Doty, 1987). In the United States 72 per cent of those over 85 are female (US National Institutes of Health, 1992, p. 8). Older women appear to receive less assistance from relatives and friends than older men of the same age, despite the fact that they suffer higher rates of certain disabling diseases, including arthritis, Alzheimer's Disease, osteoporosis and diabetes (Heikkinen *et al.*, 1983; Verbrugge, 1985).

Because of the incorporation of birth control and birthing itself into the orbit of doctors, younger women too make more use of medical services. This is not usually associated with organic pathology but reflects the growing role of medicine in the management of the 'normal' process of pregnancy and childbirth (or its prevention). Women also appear to experience more problems with their reproductive systems than men, and again this is likely to bring them into more frequent contact with the formal health care system.

Finally, evidence from across the developed world suggests that more women than men consult doctors about psychological and emotional distress. In the United Kingdom, female consultation rates with general practitioners for depression and anxiety are three times and nearly two and a half times, respectively, those of males (Office of Health Economics, 1987; UK Royal College of Practitioners, 1986). Over the course of a year one British woman in every twenty aged between 25 and 74 seeks help for emotional problems from her GP, compared with one in fifty men. There is also evidence from a range of countries that women are at least twice as likely as men to be prescribed mild tranquillisers (Ashton, 1991; Balter *et al.*, 1984).

Broadly speaking then, the picture in the developed countries is one where women live longer than men but appear 'sicker' and suffer more disability. They are ill more often than men and use more medical services. Men do not suffer such frequent illness though their health problems are more often life-threatening. But sex and gender are not the only factors influencing women's health status, as we can see if we look again at the differences between women themselves.

Even within developed countries there are major variations in the health of women in different social groups. In the United States, strokes occur twice as often in black women as in white women, and they have the highest incidence of gonorrhoea and syphilis (US National Institutes of Health, 1992, p. 13). Though black women have a lower incidence of breast cancer than white women it is significant that they are more likely to die from it (ibid.). In the United Kingdom women in the lowest social class are much more likely to experience chronic illness than their more affluent counterparts. In a national survey 46 per cent of unskilled and semi-skilled women aged between 45 and 64 reported a long-standing illness compared with 34 per cent of professional and managerial women (Bridgewood and Savage, 1993). Women in the lowest social groups were also more likely than those in the professional and managerial groups to report that illness limited their daily activities (30 per cent in comparison with 20 per cent) (ibid.).

Sickness and poverty

However it is in the poorest countries that the state of women's health is at its worst. Though some affluent women are as healthy as those in the developed countries, it is clear that millions of others live in a state of chronic debility, afflicted by the diseases of poverty and the hazards of childbearing (Jacobson, 1992; Smyke, 1991). Estimates suggest that for every one of the half million women who die of pregnancy-related causes each year, at least 16 suffer long-term damage to their health – an annual total of about eight million (Royston and Armstrong, 1989, p. 187). Reproductive tract infections are also extremely common (International Women's Health Coalition, 1991). In some African countries gonorrhoea is estimated to affect as many as 40 per cent of women (WHO, 1992). These diseases are not just distressing and disabling in themselves, but often result in chronic infection with serious effects on women's overall well-being.

Millions of women in third world countries also have to cope with the broader health consequences of poverty – communicable diseases and under-nutrition. While they risk contracting the same endemic diseases as men, both biological and social factors may increase their exposure or worsen the effects. Malaria, hepatitis and leprosy, for instance, can be especially dangerous during pregnancy, while women's responsibility for domestic tasks increases their chance of contracting water-borne diseases.

The extent of undernutrition in girls and women is dramatically documented in the incidence of anaemia. Estimates suggest that at least 44 per cent of all women in third world countries are anaemic compared with about 12 per cent in developed countries (WHO, 1992, p. 62). In India the figure is as high as 88 per cent (World Bank, 1993, p. 75). This is an important indicator of general health status, suggesting that many women are chronically debilitated, never reaching the levels of good health that most women in the first world take for granted.

In these conditions of poverty, deprivation and disruption, mental distress is clearly a major risk. Though there is little statistical evidence of its prevalence, most community surveys show a pattern similar to that of developed countries, with more women than men reporting feelings of anxiety and depression. However the pattern of treatment is very different, with many more men than women receiving psychiatric help (Paltiel, 1987). Indeed evidence from many third world countries suggests that women receive less medical treatment of all kinds than men, despite their greater need. Rural women in particular are often unable to gain access to modern services, even for obstetric care. Around 75 per cent of all births in South Asia and 62 per cent in Africa still take place without a trained health worker, compared with about 1 per cent in the developed countries (UN, 1991, p. 58). While this reflects very low levels of health spending overall, it also suggests a particular reluctance to invest in the health of women and girls.

Though female life expectancy continues to rise in most third world countries, the 'harsh decade' of the 1980s and the economic rigours of structural adjustment policies have meant deteriorating health for many women (Smyke, 1991; Vickers, 1991). The number of those who are mal-nourished has risen, resulting in an increased incidence of high-risk preg-nancies and low birth-weight babies. Diseases of poverty such as tuberculosis are re-emerging while the so-called 'diseases of affluence' are beginning to proliferate, with cancer already one of the leading causes of death for women between the ages of 25 and 35. Environmental degradation has made many women's lives harder and millions are without access to clean water or sanitation. Yet fewer resources are available to care for them. In recent years a real decline in per capita health spending has been documented in three quarters of the nations in Africa and Latin America and women appear to have been the major losers (UNICEF, 1990).

Does medicine have the answer to women's health problems?

This brief sketch has generated a wide range of questions about women's health. Why do women in most countries have a longer life expectancy than men? Why do women in some countries live nearly twice as long as those in others? Why do rates of morbidity and mortality vary between social classes and ethnic groups? Why do so many women still die in childbirth? Why do women report more sickness than men? How does their race or their culture affect women's experiences of health and health care? As we shall see, medical science can offer only limited resources either for answering these questions or for changing the reality that they represent.

The 'biomedical model'

Western medicine offers a powerful framework for describing and classifying much of the sickness afflicting individuals. Using this 'biomedical model' doctors have developed the means to prevent or cure many diseases and to alleviate the symptoms of others. However many other health problems have remained resistant to their ministrations. This has drawn increasing attention to the limitations of the conceptual schema employed by doctors and other health care providers to understand complex human phenomena. Two aspects of medical practice have come under particular scrutiny: its narrowly biological orientation and its separation of individuals from their wider social environment (Busfield, 1986, p. 28).

It is no longer appropriate (if it ever was) to categorise western medicine as a monolithic unified institution devoted only to hard science and high technology. Recent years have been marked by a revival of interest in public health and a 'humanisation' of some areas of research and clinical practice. Yet the natural sciences continue to be seen as the only 'real' basis of medicine, with attention focused predominantly on the internal workings of the human body.

Health and disease are still explained primarily through an engineering metaphor in which the body is seen as a series of separate but interdependent systems (Doyal and Doyal, 1984). Ill health is treated as the mechanical failure of some part of one or more of these systems and the medical task is to repair the damage. Within this model, the complex relationship between mind and body is rarely explored and individuals are separated from both the social and cultural contexts of their lives.

References

Ashton, H. (1991) 'Psychotropic drug prescribing for women', *British Journal of Psychiatry*, vol. 158, supplement 10, pp. 30–5.

Balter, M., Manheimer, D., Mellinger, G. *et al* (1984) 'A cross-national comparison of anti-anxiety/sedative drug use', *Current Medical Research and Opinion*, vol. 8 (supplement 4), pp. 5–18.

Blaxter, M. (1990) *Health and Lifestyles* (London: Routledge).

Bridgewood, A. and Savage, D. (1993) *General Household Survey 1991* (UK Office of Population Censuses and Surveys).

Busfield, J. (1986) *Managing Madness: changing ideas and practice* (London: Hutchinson).

Doty, P. (1987) 'Health status and health services among older women: an international perspective', *World Health Statistics Quarterly*, vol. 40, pp. 279–90.

Doyal, L. and Doyal, L. (1984) 'Western Scientific Medicine: a philosophical and political prognosis', in L. Birke and J. Silvertown (eds) *More than the Parts: biology and politics* (London: Pluto Press).

Fortney, J., Susanti, I., Gadalla, S., Salch, S., Rogers, S. and Potts, M. (1986) 'Reproductive mortality in two developing countries', *American Journal of Public Health*, vol. 76, no. 2, pp. 134–8.

Heikkinen, E., Waters, W. and Brzezinski, Z. (eds) (1983) *The Elderly in Eleven Countries – a socio medical survey* (Public Health in Europe no. 21) (Copenhagen: WHO Regional Office for Europe).

International Women's Health Coalition (1991) *Reproductive tract infections in women in the Third World: national and international policy implications* (New York: IWHC).

Jacobson, J. (1992) 'Women's health, the price of poverty', in M. Koblinsky, J. Timyan and J. Gay (eds) *The Health of Women: a global perspective* (Boulder, Co: Westview Press).

Office of Health Economics (1987) *Women's Health Today* (London: OHE).

Office of Population Censuses and Surveys (OPCS) (1986) *Occupational Mortality: Decennial Supplement, England and Wales 1979–80* (London: HMSO).

Paltiel, F. (1987) 'Women and mental health: a post Nairobi perspective', *World Health Statistics Quarterly*, vol. 40, pp. 233–66.

Paykel, E. (1991) 'Depression in women', *British Journal of Psychiatry*, vol. 158 (suppl. 10), pp. 22–9.

Rodin, J. and Ickovics, J. (1990) 'Women's health: review and research agenda as we approach the 21st century', *American Psychologist*, vol. 45, no. 9, pp. 1018–34.

Rooney, C. (1992) *Antenatal Care and Maternal Health: how effective is it?, A review of the evidence* (Geneva: WHO).

Royston, E. and Armstrong, S. (1989) *Preventing Maternal Deaths* (Geneva: World Health Organisation).

Smyke, P. (1991) *Women and Health* (London: Zed Press).

UK Royal College of General Practitioners (1986) *Morbidity Statistics from General Practice 1981–2 Third National Survey* (London: HMSO).

UNICEF (1990) *The State of the World's Children 1989* (Oxford: Oxford University Press).

United Nations (1991) 'The world's women 1970–1990: trends and statistics', *Social Statistics and Indicators*, Series, K, no. 8 (New York: UN).

United States National Institutes of Health (1992) *Opportunities for Research on Women's Health* (NIH Publication no. 92–3457) (Washington, DC: US Department of Health and Human Services).

Verbrugge, L. (1985) 'An epidemiological profile of older women' in: M. Haug, A. Ford and M. Sheafor (eds) *The Physical and Mental Health of Older Women* (New York: Springer).

Verbrugge, L. (1986) 'From sneezes to adieux: stages of health for American men and women', *Social Science and Medicine* vol. 22, no. 11, pp. 1195–212.

Vickers, J. (1991) *Women and the World Economic Crisis* (London: Zed Press).

Weissman, M. and Klerman, G. (1977) 'Sex differences and the epidemiology of depression', *Archives of General Psychiatry*, vol. 24, pp. 98–111.

Whitehead, M. (1988) *The Health Divide: inequalities in health in the 1980s* (Harmondsworth: Penguin).

World Bank (1993) *World Development Report 1993: investing in health* (Oxford: Oxford University Press).

World Health Organisation (1992) *Women's Health: across age and frontier* (Geneva: WHO).

14 You are dangerous to your health*

Robert Crawford

Ideologies of individual responsibility have always been popular among providers and academics trying to justify inequality in the utilization of medical services. During the period of rapid health sector expansion, higher morbidity and mortality rates for the poor and minorities were explained by emphasizing life-style habits, especially their health and utilization behavior. These culture of poverty explanations emphasized delay in seeking medical help, resistance, and reliance on unprofessional folk healers or advisors. As Riessman summarizes (7, p. 42):

> According to these researchers, the poor have undergone multiple negative experiences with organizational systems, leading to avoidance behaviour, lack of trust, and hence a disinclination to seek care and follow medical regimens except in dire need.

Structural barriers, such as provider resistance or unavailability of services, were rarely mentioned. Neither was lack of money often discussed except in the context of explanations for patient-dumping practices or in lobbying for government reimbursement. Now, in a period of fiscal crisis and cost control, the same higher morbidity rates and demands for more access through comprehensive national health insurance are met with a barrage of statements about the limits of medicine and the lack of appropriate health behavior. Several commentators now link overuse by the poor with their faulty health habits, and the latter are linked with ignorance. Again, education is seen as the solution; and again, the role of the providers or the insurance structure, in this case as promoters of utilization, is rarely mentioned. Previously, the poor were blamed for not using medical services enough, for relying too much on their own resources, and for undue suspicion of modern medicine. Now they are blamed for relying too much on admittedly ineffective medical services and not enough on their own resources.

*This is an extract from Crawford, R. 'You are Dangerous to Your Health: The Ideology and Politics of Victim Blaming', *International Journal of Health Services*, vol. 7, no. 4, pp. 663–80, 1977.

The various measures being adopted to reduce utilization are by now familiar: the closing or reduction in size of public hospitals; the reorganization of public hospitals to operate more like private institutions; Medicaid cuts and freezes; the dramatic failure of Medicare benefits to keep pace with increased costs so that the aged pay more out of pocket for medical services than in 1965, the year before the law became effective; rising insurance premiums, co-payments, and deductibles, along with shrinking benefits and unfavorable health insurance settlements for labor; the reorganization of private hospital services to reduce or close outpatient services and to insure reliability of payment; Health Maintenance Organizations; and the series of regulatory mechanisms designed to reduce unnecessary hospital admissions, stays, and construction.

Most important, by now it is no secret that the prospects for comprehensive national health insurance have receded behind a shield of rhetoric. When President Carter announced his new hospital cost control program in April, the *New York Times* headlined, "Action on Health Insurance May be Deferred for Years." Carter warned that, "with current inflation, the cost of any national health insurance program . . . will double in just five years." White House aides stressed that Carter's "paramount domestic goal" of balancing the budget by 1981 would probably be impossible if national health insurance were enacted. And HEW Secretary Califano argued that the proposed cost control program is a necessary precondition for the time that national health insurance "or some other system" is in place (5).

Such measures cannot be taken without risking the intensification and broadening of disillusionment, especially in a larger political context of retreat from social programs, economic recession, and disaffection from American institutions. At a time when most people still equate their perceived right to health with the right to medical treatment, and at a time when the promise of universal access to effective medical care has been held out in popular and political rhetoric for more than a decade, the need for a new ideology which can replace the mystifying power of medicine is critical. The argument is explicit. Medical benefits do not need to be expanded. What is important is health and not medicine; and health is not a right. People will not relinquish their expectations unless their belief in medicine as a panacea is broken and the value of access is replaced with a new preoccupation with boot-strapping activities aimed at controlling at-risk behaviors. In a political climate of fiscal, energy, and cost crises, self-sacrifice and self-discipline emerge as dominant themes. In lieu of rights and entitlements, education, economic sanctions, and "more studies of the American family and value system" are proposed. It is an old scenario.

The politics of diversion

Social causation of disease has several dimensions. The complexities are only beginning to be explored. The victim blaming ideology, however, inhibits that understanding and substitutes instead an unrealistic behavioral model. It both ignores what is known about human behavior and minimizes the importance of evidence about the environmental assault on health. It instructs people to be individually responsible at a time when they are becoming less capable as individuals of controlling their health environment. (8,9) Although environmental dangers are often recognized, the implication is that little can be done about an ineluctable, modern, technological, and industrial society. Life-style and environmental factors are thrown together to communicate that individuals are the primary agents in shaping or modifying the effects of their environment. Victor Fuchs, for example, while recognizing environmental factors as "also relevant," asserts that "the greatest potential for reducing coronary disease, cancer, and other major killers still lies in altering personal behavior" (3, p. 46). "Emphasizing social responsibility," he philosophizes, "can increase security, but it may be the security of the 'zoo' – purchased at the expense of freedom" (3, p. 26). Or as Whalen writes (6),

> Many of our most difficult contemporary health problems, such as cancer, heart disease and accidental injury, have a built-in behavioral component . . . *If they are to be solved at all*, we must change our style of living [emphasis added].

Nor should there be "excessive preoccupations," warns Kass, "as when cancer phobia leads to government regulations that unreasonably restrict industrial activity" (1, p. 42). Thus, the practical focus of health efforts should not be on the massive and expensive task of overhauling the environment, which, it is argued, would threaten jobs and economic growth. Instead, the important, i.e. amenable, determinants of health are behavioral, cultural, and psychological.

The diffusion of a psychological world view often reinforces the masking of social causation. Even though the psychiatric model substitutes social for natural explanations, problems still tend to be seen as amenable to change through personal transformation – with or without therapy. And with or without therapy, individuals are ultimately held responsible for their own psychological well-being. Usually, no one has to blame us for some psychological failure; we blame ourselves. Thus, psychological impairment can be just as effective as moral failing or genetic inferiority in blaming the victim and reinforcing dominant social relations (10). People are alienated, unhappy, dropouts, criminals, angry, and activists, after all, because of maladjustment to one or another psychological norm.

The ideology of individual responsibility for health lends itself to this form of psychological social control. Susceptibility to at-risk behaviors, if not a moral failing, is at least a psychological failing. New evidence relating psychological state to resistance or susceptibility to disease and accidents can and will be used to shift more responsibility to the individual. Industrial psychologists have long been employed with the intention that the best way to reduce plant accidents in lieu of costly production changes is to intervene at the individual level (11). The implication is that people make themselves sick, not only mentally but physically. If job satisfaction is important to health, people should seek more rewarding employment. Cancer is a state of mind.

In another vein, many accounts of the current disease structure in the United States link disease with affluence. The affluent society and the life-styles it has wrought, it is suggested, are the sources of the individual's degeneration and adoption of at-risk behaviors. Halberstam, for example, writes that "most Americans die of excess rather than neglect or poverty" (quoted in 4, p. 22). Knowles' warning about "sloth, gluttony, alcoholic intemperance, reckless driving, sexual frenzy and smoking" and later about "social failure" (2, pp. 2, 3) are reminiscent of a popularized conception of a decaying Rome. Thus, even though some may complain about environmental hazards, people are really suffering from over-indulgence of the good society. It is that over-indulgence which must be checked. Further, by pointing to life-styles, which are usually presented as if they reflect the problems of a homogenized, affluent society, this aspect of the ideology tends to obscure the reality of class and the impact of social inequality on health. It is compatible with the conception that people are free agents. Social structure and constraints recede amidst the abundance.

Of course, several diseases do stem from the life-styles of the more affluent. Discretionary income usually allows for excessive consumption of unhealthy products; and as Eyer (12) argues, everyone suffers in variable and specific ways from the nature of work and the conditioning of life-styles in advanced capitalist society. But are the well-established relationships between low income and high infant mortality, diseases related to poor diet and malnutrition, stress, cancer, mental illness, traumas of various kinds, and other pathologies (13–17) now to be ignored or relegated to a residual factor? While long-term inequality in morbidity and mortality is declining (18), for almost every disease and for every indicator of morbidity incidence increases as income falls (19, pp. 620–621). In some specific cases, the health gap appears to be widening (20, 21). Nonetheless, Somers reassures her readers that contemporary society is tending in the direction of homogeneity (4, p. 77):

> If poverty seems so widespread, it is at least partly because our definition of poverty is so much more generous than in the past – a generosity made possible only by the pervasive affluence and the impressive technological base upon which it rests.
>
> This point – that the current crisis is the result of progress rather than retrogression or decay – is vitally important not only as a historical fact but as a guide to problem solving in the health field as elsewhere:

Finally, by focusing on the individual instead of the economic system, the ideology performs its classical role of obscuring the class structure of work. The failure to maintain health in the workplace is attributed to some personal flaw. The more than 2.5 million people disabled by occupational accidents and diseases each year and the additional 114,000 killed (22, 23) are not explained by the hazards or pace of work as much as by the lack of sufficient caution by workers, laziness about wearing respirators or the like, psychological mal-adjustment, and even by the worker's genetic susceptibility. Correspondingly, the overworked, overstressed worker is offered TM, biofeedback, psycho-logical counseling, or some other "holistic" approach to healthy behavior change, leaving intact the structure of incentives and sanctions of employers which reward the retention of health-denying behavior.

Corporate management appears to be increasingly integrating victim blaming themes into personnel policies. Physical and especially psychological health have acquired more importance for management faced with declining productivity and expanding absenteeism. The problem for management becomes more serious with its growing dependence on high-skilled and more expensive labor, and on a more complex, integrated, and predictable produc-tion process. If "lifetime job security" becomes a priority demand of labor, employee health will become all the more important. Holding individual workers responsible for their susceptibility to illness, or for an "unproductive" psychological state, reinforces management attempts to control absenteeism and enhance productivity. Job dissatisfaction and job-induced stress (in both their psychological and physical manifestations), principal sources of absenteeism and low productivity, will become identified as life-style problems of the worker. A Conference Board report on Industry Roles in Health Care observes (24, p.12),

> Psychological stress is coming increasingly into purview of those concerned with occupational health, as a potential hazard sharing the characteristics and complexities of toxic substances – having, that is, its own threshold values, variations in individual susceptibility, and interconnections with other occupational and non-occupational factors.

Workers who are found to be "irresponsible" in maintaining their health or psychological stability, as manifest in attendance records, will face sanctions, dismissals or early retirement, rationalized as stemming from employee health problems. Simultaneously, sick day benefits will be challenged or tied to productivity considerations.

If such practices do become widespread, the facilitating device will likely be health screening. Screening potential and current employees for behavioral, attitudinal, and health purposes has already gained considerable popularity among large corporations. Among the specific advantages cited for health screening are selection "of those judged to present the least risk of unstable attendance, costly illness, poor productivity, or short tenure"; development of a "medical placement code" to match employees to jobs by health specifications; and "protection of the company against future compensation claims" (24, p. 31). In addition, screening holds out the possibility of cost savings from reduced group insurance rates. In a 1974 survey of over 800 corporations with more than 500 employees each, 71 percent of the companies gave preemployment health screening examinations to some or all new employees, compared with 63 percent ten years ago. General periodic examinations jumped from 39 to 57 percent over the same period (24). New businesses are now selling employee risk evaluations, called by one firm "health hazard appraisals." The American Hospital Association is also developing health appraisal programs for use by employers. Of course, many screening practices, such as psychological testing for appropriate work attitudes, alcoholism, or screening for mental illness records, have long been in use. The availability to employers of computerized information from health insurance companies for purposes of screening has drawn criticism from groups concerned about invasion of privacy. Women have often been asked questions during job interviews about their use of birth control, and women planning to have children continue to face barriers, especially to those jobs requiring employer investment in training.

Programs are now being expanded to screen workers for susceptibility to job hazards. Not only genetic susceptibility but also other at-risk health behaviors, such as smoking, use of alcohol, or improper diet, help legitimize screening programs. But while alerting individual workers to their suscept-ibility, these programs do not address the hazardous conditions which to some degree affect all workers. Thus, all workers may be penalized *to the extent* that such programs function to divert attention from causative conditions. To the degree that the causative agent remains, the more susceptible workers are also penalized in that they must shoulder the burden of the hazardous conditions either by looking for another, perhaps non-existent job, or, if it is permitted, by taking a risk in remaining. It is worth noting in this regard that some women of childbearing age barred from working in plants using lead are reported to be obtaining sterilizations in order to regain their jobs. *Dollars and Sense* summarizes one labor leader's remarks on industry's tactics (25, p. 15):

> At a recent UAW conference on lead, UAW President Leonard Woodcock summed up industry's response to hazard control as "fix the worker, not the workplace." He voiced particular concern over exclusion of so-called "sensitive" groups of workers, the use of dangerous chemical agents to artificially lower workers' blood lead levels, the transfer of workers in and out of high lead areas, and the forced use of personal respirators instead of engineering controls to clean the air in the workplace.

Thus, whether or not the individual is personally blamed for some at-risk behavior, excluding the "susceptible" worker from the workplace is like asking "vulnerable" people to reduce activity during an ozone watch: it may be helpful for particular individuals, but under the guise of health promotion, it may also act as a colossal masquerade.

Some related issues

It is important to recognize and address the issue that a significant portion of socially caused illness is, at some level, associated with individual, at-risk behavior which can be changed to improve health. A deterministic view which argues that individuals have no choice should be avoided. What must be questioned is both the effectiveness and the political uses (as well as the scientific narrowness) of a focus on life-styles and on changing individual behavior without changing the social and economic environment. Just as the Horatio Alger myth was based on the fact that just enough individuals achieve mobility to make believable the possibility, significant health gains are clearly realizable for those who just try hard enough to resist the incredible array of social forces aligned against healthy behavior. McKinlay has convincingly argued that the frequent failure of health education programs designed to change individual behavior is attributable to the failure to address the social context. In reviewing some of the strategies adopted by the "manufacturers of illness" to encourage profitable at-risk behaviors and to shape conducive self-images in American consumers, McKinlay observes that (26, pp. 9–10):

> . . . certain at-risk behaviors have become so inextricably intertwined with our dominant cultural system (perhaps even symbolic of it) that the routine display of such behavior almost signifies membership in this society . . . To request people to change or alter these behaviors is more or less to request the abandonment of dominant culture.

Certainly, the development of health education programs should be encouraged. Concurrent with expansion of access to primary medical services, health personnel should be trained to work with patients in developing practices which reduce risk factors. Lack of information about the dangers of smoking, high cholesterol intake, or obesity, for example, could be considerably reduced by such efforts. The solid evidence supporting Belloc and Breslow's (27) prescriptions for a healthier and longer life could be made available. Health educators, however, would be engaging in victim blaming if such efforts were allowed to suffice; and only marginal results would be achieved as well.

References

1 Kass, L. Regarding the end of medicine and the pursuit of health. *Public Interest* No. 40: 11–42, summer 1975.
2 *Conference on Future Directions in Health Care: The Dimensions of Medicine.* Sponsored by the Blue Cross Association, The Rockefeller Foundation, and Health Policy Program, University of California, New York, December 1975.
3 Fuchs, V. *Who Shall Live? Health, Economics, and Social Choice.* Basic Books, New York, 1974.
4 Somers, A. *Health Care in Transition: Directions for the Future.* Hospital Research and Educational Trust, Chicago, 1971.

5 *New York Times*, April 26, 1977.

6 *New York Times*, April 17, 1977.

7 Riessman, C. K. The use of health services by the poor. *Social Policy* 5(1): 41–49, 1974.

8 Special Issue on the Economy, Medicine, and Health, edited by Joseph Eyer. *Int. J. Health Serv.* 7(1): 1–150, 1977.

9 The Social Etiology of Disease (Part I). *HMO-A Network for Marxist Studies in Health* No. 2, January 1977.

10 Edelman, M. The political language of the helping professions. *Politics and Society* 4(3): 295–310, 1974.

11 *New York Times*, April 3, 1977.

12 Eyer, J. Prosperity as a cause of disease. *Int. J. Health Serv.* 7(1): 125–150, 1977.

13 Hurley, R. The health crisis of the poor. In *The Social Organization of Health*, edited by H. P. Dreitzel, pp. 83–122. Macmillan Company, New York, 1971.

14 *Infant Mortality Rates: Socioeconomic Factors*, Series 22, No. 14. U.S. Public Health Service, Washington, D.C., 1972.

15 *Selected Vital and Health Statistics in Poverty and Nonpoverty Areas of 19 Large Cities, United States, 1969–71*, Series 21, No. 26. U.S. Public Health Service, Washington, D.C., 1975.

16 Kitagawa, E. and Hauser, P. *Differential Mortality in the United States: A Study in Socio-economic Epidemiology*. Harvard University Press, Cambridge, 1973.

17 Sherer, H. Hypertension. *HMO-A Network for Marxist Studies in Health* No. 2, January 1977.

18 Antonovsky, A. Social class, life expectancy, and overall mortality. *Milbank Mem. Fund Q.* 45(2, part I): 31–73, 1967.

19 *Preventive Medicine USA*. Prodist, New York, 1976.

20 Jenkins, C. D. Recent evidence supporting psychologic and social risk factors for coronary heart diseases. *N. Engl. J. Med.* 294(18): 987–994, 1976, and 294(19): 1033–1038, 1976.

21 Eyer, J. and Sterling, P. Stress related mortality and social organization. *Review of Radical Political Economy*, forthcoming.

22 Page, J. A. and O'Brien, M. *Bitter Wages*. Grossman Publishers, New York, 1973.

23 Brodeur, P. *Expendable Americans*. Viking Press, New York, 1974.

24 Lusterman, S. *Industry Roles in Health Care*. The Conference Board, Inc., New York, 1974.

25 *Dollars and Sense*, April 1977.

26 McKinlay, J. A. Case for Refocussing Upstream – The Political Economy of Illness. Unpublished paper, Boston University, 1974.

27 Belloc, N. B. and Breslow, L. Relationship of physical health status and health practices. *Prev. Med.* 1(3): 409–421, 1972.

15 Beyond the Black Report*

*Mel Bartley, David Blane and
George Davey Smith*

Structure and agency

The classic sociological problem of structure and agency is well exemplified in this collection. Health inequality research needs to acknowledge that it is not just the nature of the social environment, but its dynamics which must be understood. Modern industrial economies work by getting at least some people to produce more than the value of the wages they are paid. This surplus is retained by employers (or ruling bureaucracies) and forms the basis of profit, the driving mechanism of the economic system. The fact that some citizens are poorer than others is therefore not an accident of bad planning or even individual greed. The reason for increasing numbers of 'excluded' people in late 20th century advanced industrial society is the increasing power of technology to produce ever more goods with ever fewer human workers. One result is 'social exclusion'. Like the Native Americans in the 19th century (Higgs and Scambler 1998), the traditional (especially male) working class is becoming surplus to economic requirements in the late 20th century. The native American people were confined to reservations and granted small amounts of land and welfare payments: significantly the destruction of their communities was brought about in its later phases not by overt genocide but by the health consequences of utter demoralisation. Although inequality may take new forms, the chapters in this book show the implausibility of the idea that 'class has disappeared'. They add to the evidence of large social differences in quality of residential environment, political attitudes, voting, car and home ownership as well as the very different patterns of educational and career attainment among children from different social backgrounds. People from mining areas may no longer wear cloth caps, but the waning of stereotyped cultural signals co-exists with a wide belief that class distinction is alive and well in Britain today (Marshall *et al.* 1988).

Popay and her colleagues criticise the concentration of many studies of health inequality on individuals' 'risk factors' and 'risk behaviour' to the

*This is an extract from Bartley, M., Blane, D., Davey Smith, G. 'Introduction: beyond the Black Report', *Sociology of Health & Illness*, vol. 20, no. 5. pp. 563–77, 1998.

relative neglect of the macrosocial environment. However, they also call for greater understanding at the micro level. They take up a question implicit in the essay of Wilkinson and Kawachi: why is it that people located within the social structures where we find them behave in the way they do? The continuity of social structure is itself produced by myriad individual decisions and actions. Most people who decide whether or not to take a school exam or aim for promotion at work are not consciously reproducing the class system: they are doing what seems best to them at the time. Similarly most people lighting up a cigarette or going out jobbing are not aiming to reproduce the pattern of health inequality. Once health education has disseminated information about the risks of behaviours such as smoking and inadequate diet, we still need some explanation of why those in the most socially disadvantaged positions seem least able to adopt healthier lifestyles; studies show that they are equally willing to do so (Lee *et al.* 1991).

We understand very little about these patterns of decision and action, perhaps in part because of the neglect of agency criticised by Popay *et al.* The UK Economic and Social Research Council's recent initiative in funding a programme of work on Social Variations in Health will help to overcome this lack. Several of the projects funded by the programme, including ones in which Shaw and Popay and their collaborators are involved, are concentrating on an ethnographic approach, placing the researchers in the communities identified by geographical studies as having poor health, and collecting face to face data on attitudes, actions and ideas of residents. This is probably the largest amount of resources ever devoted to ethnographic study of health inequality. Hopefully in a few years, a collection of ethnographic work on the meaning of inequality in everyday life will be put together. A particularly valuable product of this research could be an increased understanding of how position in a social hierarchy may influence health in the way postulated by Wilkinson and others.

If we are to direct attention simultaneously to structure and agency, then studies of delimited areas become necessary: neighbourhoods are where individuals do encounter social structure and live out life-courses. At this point the concept of 'social capital' becomes relevant to the debate on health inequality. What is the effect on individual deprivation of the quality of social relationships? Perhaps we can discuss the concept by beginning with William Farr's formula for predicting area differences in mortality (Eyler 1979). Farr regarded the excess mortality (over and above the 'ideal' rate) in an area as determined by hygienic conditions (crowding and the 'number of germs in the atmosphere') only where the average income was greater than or equal to the price of 'necessities'. '[O]nly where [the market price of all necessities of life in an area] is greater than [the average wage] did low income exert an important influence on mortality. Under other conditions, hygiene was more important' (Eyler 1979: 126). The poorer the inhabitants, the more important was hygiene. Today some health inequality researchers might substitute 'social capital' for 'hygiene' in this model: where income is sufficient to cover bare necessities, population health depends on social cohesion. However, successive attempts to determine the real cost of the minimum basic necessities of life have conspicuously failed (Veit-Wilson 1992). Living standards are subject to a 'historical and moral component' which depends on the cost of symbolic goods needed for full social participation as well as physical subsistence (Bartley 1991). For example, where do such goods as education and health care come in this equation? In the post war welfare state these were provided as part of the social wage: now their quality, if not availability, increasingly depends on individual income. It may well be that where public provision for schools and health services is declining, the social composition of an area may make up for declining levels of social wage, that is, instead of the density of germs in the air, we would take the density of 'social capital'.

For example, consider the different performance of children in comprehensive schools according to the social makeup of the catchment area (Morris *et al.* 1996). Morris and colleagues found that an index of local social conditions was significantly related both to average school attainment and to local mortality rates. This ecological analysis seemed to indicate that there was some characteristic of localities which affected both the school attainment of children and the life expectancy of their elders. It is a commonplace among middle class parents in urban areas that the social composition of the school will affect the burden on a school's teachers (Buchel and Duncan 1998). What is happening is that the better-off children's families are subsidising (in terms of social support and unpaid domestic labour) the efforts of the teachers by sending out children who are already well socialised, able to read, etc. This allows more time and effort to be devoted to the less fortunate children. But surely the same will be true of all socially provided services. Because more of the overhead costs of health maintenance of middle class workers are carried by employers, in terms of sick pay, longer holidays, paid time off to visit the doctor etc., there are shorter hospital waiting lists in middle class than working class residential areas, which will of course mean that even poorer people in wealthy areas wait less long for medical care. This is not, however, the way in which 'social capital' is usually expressed (Messer 1998, Moser 1998, Woolcock 1998). It is more usually taken to be the density of social relationships amongst local residents, with the implication that higher levels of communication and support between individuals adds to the common good (Putnam *et al.* 1993, 1995: 664–5 cited in Wilkinson 1996). It is the contention of 'communitarianism', at least implicitly, that in a re-moralised society fewer public resources would be needed, for example, to support parents, elderly people and those who are chronically ill, as this would be done by 'the community', as part of solidaristic commitment, without cost to the employer or the state. Even the cost of goods for individual consumption, and thereby the income/necessities ratio, would, in this view, be lowered by high levels of social capital, thus enabling a lower wage to cover the reproduction costs of labour power.

But what is it that links social conditions, however they are characterised, to the health of the individual? A message common to the chapters by

Wilkinson and Kawachi and Popay and her colleagues, and shared by the wider literature on emotions and the body, is the importance of personal identity. One thing researchers are starting to ask is: What resources does each social form make available to individuals from which they may shape an identity they can live with? These considerations are most acute in the literature on disability; but they may also turn out to be crucial for health inequality research as a whole. Future research may well set out to discover how action is shaped by the narratives people construct to make sense of their own encounters with inequality. One strategy which has been well described in the literature on illness behaviour is that known as 'normalis-ation': rather than bear the threat to self-esteem inherent in the admission of a problem, many will find skillful ways to deny it. Improved under-standing of an important source of the persistence of health inequality may well lie in the sensitive analysis of such strategies of denying the existence of subordination.

Curtis and Jones take up the issue of how to study health inequality in localities, but give more attention to the quantitative methods which have been used in existing studies. Saying that the locality is where individuals encounter social structure and the agency of others is all very well; however, evidence for an 'area effect' independent of individual characteristics remains elusive and contradictory. Some might be wary of the danger that the dynamics of class society might once again be forgotten in the attempt to show that policies to increase 'social capital' in neighbourhoods could overcome sharp inequalities in individual living standards (Sloggett and Joshi 1994). To say that structure and agency operate to a large extent in face to face local encounters is one thing, to claim that there are 'area effects' which might attenuate or exacerbate health inequality is quite another. As Curtis and Jones point out, policy implications of such research need to be drawn with great caution. Although the question of social capital, now rising up the health policy agenda, is not directly addressed in this book, the authors of several of the chapters take valuable steps towards clarifying an intellectual context for future work on this topic.

Social and spatial inequalities in health

The second part of this collection assembles a set of empirical studies of health inequality in Britain and the Netherlands at the end of the 20th century. Given the richness of health inequality research at the present time, these inevitably cover only part of the full spectrum. Cameron and Bernardes take a refreshing stance in that they problematise men's, rather than women's health behaviour; a perspective that has been rather lacking given the lower life expectancy of men in most developed industrial societies. Their paper's concern with the barriers to seeking treatment for prostate problems allows them to open up the whole area of 'male embodiment' at a time of rapid change in gender roles, and its implications for health policy.

A gap in the collection might appear to be an essay specifically dealing with policy. However, most of the chapters can clearly be seen to have emerged from policy concerns, even if some of these are at a more 'macro' level than health or social planning in individual nations. At a time of such rapid change, authors seem to have concluded that what is more important is to establish a firm base in terms of theory and observation rather than jump towards policy prescriptions too soon. The contribution of Shaw and her colleagues takes up the call made in some of the theoretical chapters for work on health differences between geographical areas, and shows new data on increases in health inequality. Whereas previous literature has concentrated on increasing differences between officially defined social classes (Drever and Whitehead 1997) or a limited number of areas (McLoone and Boddy 1994, McCarron *et al.*, Phillimore *et al.* 1994). Shaw *et al.* show how mortality differences between more and less disadvantaged areas are now at the highest level ever recorded. Once again, the authors relate their findings to policy debate in a thoughtful discussion which sets out their uncertainty as to the interpretation of these findings, and offers suggestions as to how research might address these uncertainties.

Throughout the book, there is an unpacking of traditional social classifications. 'Male gender' is shown by Cameron and Bernardes' rich qualitative material to be many-faceted and to allow a wide variety of responses to the threats posed by chronic illness. Nazroo emphasises the importance of theoretical approaches to the definitions of 'class' and 'ethnicity', and shows the dangers that arise for empirical studies when untheorised definitions are accepted uncritically. He shows how crude and inappropriate measures of inequality can lead to an apparent failure of structural explanations for ethnic differences in health. This, in turn, has led, in some studies, to appeals either to genetic or cultural interpretation of health differences between ethnic groups by a process of elimination. His chapter provides a striking instance of how policy prescriptions based on the use of stereotypical social categories can be seriously misleading. His own development of meaningful categories for the study of health inequality among ethnic minority groups returns to basic considerations of structure and agency, showing that even within the same social classes, members of such groups experienced lower paid, less prestigious and more stressful work, greater job insecurity, and longer periods of unemployment. Both theoretical (Kauffman *et al.* 1997) and empirical (Davey Smith *et al.* 1998) work from the United States has framed questions regarding the association of ethnicity and socioeconomic position in a similar way. The practice of treating class as a 'variable' rather than as part of a set of social relations is increasingly criticised both in the USA (Krieger *et al.* 1997), and in Britain (Higgs and Scambler 1998). Nazroo's paper shows how this results in the failure to capture inequality among ethnic minority citizens, not because the sources of this inequality are genetic or cultural, but because it misrepresents their material situation.

Burrows and Nettleton focus on housing insecurity, an experience which affected people from many different social backgrounds during the 1980s and early 1990s. Their scene-setting, describing the changes in both the labour market and the housing market during the 1980s, forms an invaluable context for all the other papers based on UK data. Their description of mortgage indebtedness as most often a part of a general 'struggle to keep one's health above water' is a striking exemplification of the 'accumulation of risk' theory now growing in importance in health inequality research (Blane *et al.* 1993, Davey Smith *et al.* 1994, Kreiger 1994, Blane 1995, Wunsch *et al.* 1996). Their qualitative data echo much of what has been discussed in the papers by Wilkinson and Kawachi and Elstad: the importance of social honour and the role played by material goods such as a privately owned house in maintaining this sometimes fragile state. They relate this to questions of identity and biographical disruption (Bury 1982). In this way, an empirical paper adds yet more to the complex picture of the relationships between social forms and individual well-being and sets an example of how to bring general notions about 'social inequality' down to earth in ways that offer plausible pathways to health effects.

Perhaps the most important development in health inequality research in the recent past has been the opening out of a new perspective (though one which was anticipated by mid-century social medicine): the importance of the lifecourse. In 1994 the UK government (then a Conservative one) set up a committee of inquiry into 'social variation in health' (*British Medical Journal* 1994) (the Metters committee) which, in its report, took a quietly revolutionary step. It passed beyond the post-Black Report framework of explanations for health inequality, spending little or no time on the discussion of artifact or selection explanations (Variations sub-group 1995). While accepting that the determinants of health inequality arose from the structure of society and its influences on individual lifestyle and quality of life, the Metters Report went on to acknowledge the importance of how these influences work over time.

The Black Report had, of course, itself put emphasis in its policy proposals on improving the circumstances of children, because, as it said, early life 'casts long shadows forward' onto the health of the adult. The founders of the British cohort studies must to some extent have foreseen the importance of early life for adult health. What could not have been foreseen, however, was the extent to which a lifecourse approach would offer the solution to the problem of combining the findings relating to social inequality with those relating to individual living standards and the observed fine grain of health inequality. The more data we have which show, as do those presented here by van de Mheen and her colleagues, how early circumstances contribute to health in later life, the clearer it becomes that 'social class' at any given point is but a very partial indicator of a whole sequence, a 'probabilistic cascade' of events which need to be seen in combination if the effects of social environment on health are to be understood (Blane *et al.* 1996, Davey Smith *et al.* 1997). Different individuals have arrived at any particular level of income, occupational advantage or prestige with different life histories behind them. Variables such as height, education, and ownership of additional consumer goods act as indicators of these past histories. Those with the greatest accumulation of 'bio-material' advantages are likely to have experienced optimal combinations of events from childhood onwards. Hence the fine grain – the two cars and the rather large house – are serving to indicate that bit more financial security throughout the life of the individual, or in their extended family, as anyone who remembers which students had cars as undergraduates will perhaps recognise. The significance of the degree of inequality in a society is that this indicates how severe the longer term implications of any given adverse event as the life course unfolds is likely to be (unemployment or illness of the bread winner, marital breakdown, periods of under-achievement at school or in the early work career, etc.) and how likely it is to set off a descending spiral of other disadvantages (Power and Matthews 1997; Kuh *et al.* 1997)

References

Bartley, M. (1991) Health and labour force participation: stress, selection and the reproduction costs of labour power. *Journal of Social Policy*, 21, 327–64.

Blane, D. (1995) Social determinants of health – socioeconomic status, social class and ethnicity. *American Journal of Public Health*, 85, 903–4.

Blane, D., Davey Smith, G. and Bartley, M. (1993) Social selection: what does it contribute to social class differences in health? *Sociology of Health and Illness*, 15, 1–15.

Blane, D., Hart, C.L., Davey Smith, G., Gillis, C.R., Hole, D.J. and Hawthorne, V.M. (1996) Association of cardiovascular disease risk factors with socioeconomic position during childhood and during adulthood. *British Medical Journal*, 313, 1434–8.

British Medical Journal (1994) British government looks at effects of wealth on health. *British Medical Journal*, 308, 1257.

Buchel, F. and Duncan, G.J. (1998) Do parents' social activities promote children's school attainment? Evidence from the German socioeconomic panel. *Journal of Marriage and the Family*, 60, 95–108.

Bury, M.R. (1982) Chronic illness as biographical disruption. *Sociology of Health and Illness*, 4, 2, 167–82.

Davey Smith, G., Blane, D. and Bartley, M. (1994) Explanations for socio-economic differentials in mortality: evidence from Britain and elsewhere. *European Journal of Public Health*, 4, 131–44.

Davey Smith, G., Hart, C., Blane, D., Gillis, C. and Hawthorne, V. (1997) Lifetime socioeconomic position and mortality: prospective observational study. *British Medical Journal*, 314, 547–52.

Davey Smith, G., Neaton, J.D., Wentworth, D. and Stamler, R. (1998) Mortality differences between black and white men in the USA: contribution of income and other risk factors among men screened for the MRFIT. *Lancet*, 351, 934–9.

Drever, F. and Whitehead, M. (1977) *Health Inequalities*. London: HMSO.

Eyler, J. (1979) *William Farr and Victorian Social Medicine*. Baltimore: Johns Hopkins University Press.

Higgs, P. and Scambler, G. (1998) Explaining health inequalities: how useful are concepts of social class? In Higgs, P. and Scambler, G. (eds) *Modernity, Medicine and Health*. London: Routledge.

Kauffman, J.S., McGee, D.L. and Cooper, R.S. (1997) Socioeconomic status and health in blacks and whites: the problem of residual confounding and the resiliency of race. *Epidemiology*, 8, 621–8.

Kreiger, N. (1994) Epidemiology and the web of causation: has anyone seen the spider? *Social Science and Medicine*, 39, 887–903.

Krieger, N., Williams, D.R. and Moss, N.E. (1997) Measuring social class in US public health research: concepts, methodologies and guidelines. *Annual Review of Public Health*, 18, 341–78.

Kuh, D.J.L., Power, C., Blane, D. and Bartley, M. (1997) Social pathways between childhood and adult health. In Kuh, D.J.L. and Ben Shlomo, Y. (eds) *Lifecourse Approach to Chronic Disease Epidemiology*, Oxford: Oxford University Press.

Lee, A.J., Crombie, I.L.K., Smith, W.C.S. and Tunstall-Pedoe, H.D. (1991) Cigarette smoking and employment status. *Social Science and Medicine*, 32, 1309–12.

Marshall, G., Newby, H., Rose, D. and Volger, C. (1988) *Social Class in Modern Britain*. London: Hutchinson.

McCarron, P.G., Davey Smith, G. and Womersley, J.J. (1994) Deprivation and mortality in Glasgow: changes from 1980 to 1992. *British Medical Journal*, 309, 1481–2.

McLoone, P. and Boddy, A. (1994) Deprivation and mortality in Scotland, 1981 and 1991. *British Medical Journal*, 309, 1465–70.

Messer, J. (1988) Agency, communication, and the formation of social capital. *Nonprofit and Voluntary Sector Quarterly*, 27, 5–12.

Morris, J.N., Blane, D.B. and White, I.R. (1996) Levels of mortality, education and social conditions in the 107 local education authority areas of England. *Journal of Epidemiology and Community Health*, 50, 15–17.

Moser, C.O.N. (1998) The asset vulnerability framework: reassessing urban poverty reduction strategies. *World Developments*, 26, 1–19.

Phillimore, P., Beattie, A. and Townsend, P. (1994) Widening inequality of health in northern England, 1981–91. *British Medical Journal*, 308, 1125–8.

Power, C. and Matthews, S. (1997) Origins of health inequalities in a national population sample. *Lancet*, 350, 1584–9.

Putnam, R.D. (1995) Tuning in, tuning out: the strange disappearance of social capital in America. *Political Science and Politics*, 4, 664–83.

Putnam, R.D., Leonardi, R. and Nanetti, R.Y. (1993) *Making Democracy Work: Civic Tradition in Modern Italy*. Princeton, NJ: Princeton University Press.

Sloggett, A. and Joshi, H. (1994) Higher mortality in deprived areas: community or personal disadvantage? *British Medical Journal*, 309, 1470–4.

Variations Sub-group of the Chief Medical Officer's Health of the Nation Working Group (1995) *Variations in Health: What can the Department of Health and the NHS Do?* London: Department of Health.

Veit Wilson, J. (1992) Muddle or mendacity – the Beveridge Committee and the poverty line. *Journal of Social Policy*, 21, 269–301.

Wilkinson, R.G. (1996) *Unhealthy Societies: the Afflictions of Inequality*. London: Routledge.

Woolcock, M. (1998) Social capital and economic development: toward a theoretical synthesis and policy framework. *Theory and Society*, 27, 151–208.

Wunsch, D., Duchène, J., Thilgès, E. and Salhi, M. (1996) Socio-economic differences in mortality: a lifecourse approach. *European Journal of Population*, 12, 167–85.

16 The Acheson Report*

Sir Donald Acheson (Chairman)

Our task has been to review the evidence on inequalities in health in England, including time trends, and, as a contribution to the development of the Government's strategy for health, to identify areas for policy development likely to reduce these inequalities. We carried out our task over the last 12 months, drawing on scientific and expert evidence, and peer review.

Although average mortality has fallen over the past 50 years, unacceptable inequalities in health persist. For many measures of health, inequalities have either remained the same or have widened in recent decades.

These inequalities affect the whole of society and they can be identified at all stages of the life course from pregnancy to old age.

The weight of scientific evidence supports a socioeconomic explanation of health inequalities. This traces the roots of ill health to such determinants as income, education and employment as well as to the material environment and lifestyle. It follows that our recommendations have implications across a broad front and reach far beyond the remit of the Department of Health. Some relate to the whole Government while others relate to particular Departments.

We have identified a range of ideas for future policy development, judged on the scale of their potential impact on health inequalities, and the weight of evidence. These areas include: poverty, income, tax and benefits; education; employment; housing and environment; mobility, transport and pollution; and nutrition. Areas are also identified by the stages of the life course – mothers, children and families; young people and adults of working age; and older people – and by focusing on ethnic and gender inequalities. We identify possible steps within the National Health Service to reduce inequalities. In our view, these areas offer opportunities over time to improve the health of the less well off.

There are three areas which we regard as crucial:

*This is an abridged extract from Sir Donald Acheson (Chairman) (1998) *Independent Inquiry into Inequalities in Health Report*, The Stationery Office, pp. xi, 5–9, 29–30, 120–24, 129–30.

- all policies likely to have an impact on health should be evaluated in terms of their impact on health inequalities;
- a high priority should be given to the health of families with children;
- further steps should be taken to reduce income inequalities and improve the living standards of poor households. [. . .]

Socioeconomic model of health

We have adopted a socioeconomic model of health and its inequalities. This is in line with the weight of scientific evidence. Figure 1 shows the main determinants of health as layers of influence, one over another.[1,2] At the centre are individuals, endowed with age, sex and constitutional factors which undoubtedly influence their health potential, but which are fixed. Surrounding the individuals are layers of influence that, in theory, could be modified. The innermost layer represents the personal behaviour and way of life adopted by individuals, containing factors such as smoking habits and physical activity, with the potential to promote or damage health. But individuals do not exist in a vacuum: they interact with friends, relatives and their immediate community, and come under the social and community influences represented in the next layer. Mutual support within a community can sustain the health of its members in otherwise unfavourable conditions. The wider influences on a person's ability to maintain health (shown in the third layer) include their

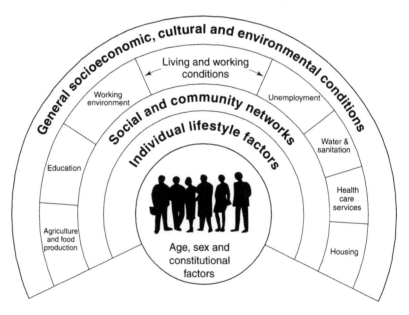

Figure 1 The main determinants of health.

Source: Dahlgren G. and Whitehead M. (1991)[1]

living and working conditions, food supplies and access to essential goods and services. Overall there are the economic, cultural and environmental conditions prevalent in society as a whole, represented in the outermost layer.

The model emphasises interactions between these different layers. For example, individual lifestyles are embedded in social and community networks and in living and working conditions, which in turn are related to the wider cultural and socioeconomic environment.

Socioeconomic inequalities in health reflect differential exposure – from before birth and across the life span – to risks associated with socioeconomic position. These differential exposures are also important in explaining health inequalities which exist by ethnicity and gender.

This model has been used to guide research. The research task is to trace the paths from social structure, represented by socioeconomic status, through to inequalities in health. This can be done in stages, for example showing that work is related to pathophysiological changes such as raised blood pressure or biochemical disturbances which are in turn related to disease risk; or showing that the social environment in which people live is related to their health behaviour, such as patterns of eating, drinking, smoking and physical activity.

The model also illustrates various intervention points. Medical care, for example, might intervene at the level of morbidity to prevent progression to death, or earlier, at the level of pathophysiological changes to interrupt transition to morbidity.

Preventive approaches might act at the level of attempting to change individual risk, by encouraging people to give up smoking or change diet. Interventions in the workplace or the social environment might encourage a climate which promotes healthy behaviour or improved psychological conditions. Interventions at the level of social structure would reduce social and economic inequalities.

Our approach is shared by the Government which, in "Our Healthier Nation", has expressed its determination to tackle "*the root causes of health*". The Prime Minister emphasised this approach in his answer to a Parliamentary Question on low income, inequality and health (11th June 1997).

". . . It is for that reason that the Secretary of State for Health has asked Sir Donald Acheson to conduct a further review into inequality and the link between health and wealth . . . These inequalities do matter and there is no doubt that the published statistics show a link between income, inequality and poor health. It is important to address that issue, and we are doing so. The purpose of the windfall tax is to address that matter on behalf of young people and the long-term unemployed. We are also addressing the issue by introducing the minimum wage, which will help those on low incomes, and with welfare measures, particularly those designed to get single parents back to work".[3]

Need to intervene on a broad front

The socioeconomic model also dictates the breadth of our review. A broad front approach reflects scientific evidence that health inequalities are the outcome of causal chains which run back into and from the basic structure of society. Such an approach is also necessary because many of the factors are interrelated. It is likely to be less effective to focus solely on one point if complementary action is not in place which influences a linked factor in another policy area. Policies need to be both "upstream" and "downstream".

For instance, a policy which reduces inequalities in income and improves the income of the less well off, and one which provides pre-school education for all four year olds are examples of "upstream" policies which are likely to have a wide range of consequences, including benefits to health. Policies such as providing nicotine replacement therapy on prescription, or making available better facilities for taking physical exercise, are "downstream" interventions which have a narrower range of benefits.

We have, therefore, recommended both "upstream" and "downstream" policies – those which deal with wider influences on health inequalities such as income distribution, education, public safety, housing, work environment, employment, social networks, transport and pollution, as well as those which have narrower impacts, such as on healthy behaviours. [. . .]

Priority for parents and children

While remediable risk factors affecting health occur throughout the life course, childhood is a critical and vulnerable stage where poor socioeconomic circumstances have lasting effects. Follow up through life of successive samples of births has pointed to the crucial influence of early life on subsequent mental and physical health and development.[4] The fact that the adverse outcomes, for example, mental illness, short stature, obesity, delinquency and unemployment, cover a wide range, carries an important message. It suggests that policies which reduce such early adverse influences may result in multiple benefits, not only throughout the life course of that child but to the next generation.

Another line of research, which concentrates on the effects of a mother's nutrition on her child's later health, has shown that small size or thinness at birth are associated with coronary heart disease, diabetes and hypertension in later life. As two principal determinants of a baby's weight at birth are the mother's pre-pregnant weight and her own birthweight, the need for policies to improve the health of (future) mothers and their children is obvious.[5] It also follows that, among migrants who move from a poorly nourished to a well nourished community, there will be implications for fetal growth and adult health for more than one generation.

Taking into account these findings and the view expressed in "Our Healthier Nation" that "*good health is the supreme gift parents can give their children*", we take the view that, while there are many potentially beneficial interventions to reduce inequalities in health in adults of working age and older people, many of those with the best chance of reducing future inequalities in mental and physical health relate to parents, particularly present and future mothers, and children. [. . .]

Cross-Government issues

If future inequalities in health are to be reduced, it will be essential to carry out a wide range of policies to achieve both a general improvement in health and a greater impact on the less well off. By this we mean those who in terms of socioeconomic status, gender or ethnicity are less well off than average in terms of health or its principal determinants – such as income, education, employment or the material environment.

The impact of policies designed to improve health may have different consequences for different groups of people which are not always appreciated. Some policies will both improve health and reduce health inequalities. The introduction of the NHS benefited the health of all sections of the population, particularly women and children, many of whom were excluded from previous arrangements under the National Insurance Act.

A well intended policy which improves average health may have no effect on inequalities. It may even widen them by having a greater impact on the better off. Classic examples include policies aimed at preventing illness, if they resulted in uptake favouring the better off. This has happened in some initiatives concerned with immunisation and cervical screening, as well as in some campaigns to discourage smoking or to promote breastfeeding. More recently, the Government's welcome decision to provide a pre-school place for every child aged four in the country is likely to benefit health on average but could have the unintended effect of increasing inequalities. This would happen if the children of the better off made more effective use of the service.

These examples highlight the need for extra attention to the needs of the less well off. This could be accommodated both by policies directed at the least well off and by an approach which would require the need for inequalities to be addressed wherever universal services are provided, such as publicly funded education and the National Health Service, and where other policies are likely to have an impact on health.

A broader approach of this kind which explicitly addresses inequalities could provide a new direction for public policy. It is our view that, in general, reductions in inequalities are most likely to be achieved if policies are formulated with the reduction of inequalities in mind. [. . .]

List of recommendations

General recommendations

1   We RECOMMEND that as part of health impact assessment, all policies likely to have a direct or indirect effect on health should be

evaluated in terms of their impact on health inequalities, and should be formulated in such a way that by favouring the less well off they will, wherever possible, reduce such inequalities.

1.1   We recommend establishing mechanisms to monitor inequalities in health and to evaluate the effectiveness of measures taken to reduce them.

1.2   We recommend a review of data needs to improve the capacity to monitor inequalities in health and their determinants at a national and local level.

2   We RECOMMEND a high priority is given to policies aimed at improving health and reducing health inequalities in women of childbearing age, expectant mothers and young children.

Poverty, income, tax and benefits

3   We RECOMMEND policies which will further reduce income inequalities, and improve the living standards of households in receipt of social security benefits. Specifically:

3.1   we recommend further reductions in poverty in women of childbearing age, expectant mothers, young children and older people should be made by increasing benefits in cash or in kind to them.

3.2   We recommend uprating of benefits and pensions according to principles which protect and, where possible, improve the standard of living of those who depend on them and which narrow the gap between their standard of living and average living standards

3.3   We recommend measures to increase the uptake of benefits in entitled groups.

Education

4   We RECOMMEND the provision of additional resources for schools serving children from less well off groups to enhance their educational achievement. The Revenue Support Grant formula and other funding mechanisms should be more strongly weighted to reflect need and socioeconomic disadvantage.

5   We RECOMMEND the further development of high quality pre-school education so that it meets, in particular, the needs of disadvantaged families. We also recommend that the benefits of pre-school education to disadvantaged families are evaluated and, if necessary, additional resources are made available to support further development.

6   We RECOMMEND the further development of "health promoting schools", initially focused on, but not limited to, disadvantaged communities.

7   We RECOMMEND further measures to improve the nutrition provided at school, including: the promotion of school food policies;

the development of budgeting and cooking skills; the preservation of free school meals entitlement; the provision of free school fruit; and the restriction of less healthy food.

Employment

8   We RECOMMEND policies which improve the opportunities for work and which ameliorate the health consequences of unemployment. Specifically:

8.1 we recommend further steps to increase employment opportunities.

8.2 We recommend further investment in high quality training for young and long-term unemployed people.

We recommend policies which will further reduce income inequalities, and improve the living standards of households in receipt of social security benefits (recommendation 3).

We recommend an integrated policy for the provision of affordable, high quality day care and pre-school education with extra resources for disadvantaged communities (recommendation 21.1).

9   We RECOMMEND policies to improve the quality of jobs, and reduce psychosocial work hazards. Specifically:

9.1 we recommend employers, unions and relevant agencies take further measures to improve health through good management practices which lead to an increased level of control, variety and appropriate use of skills in the workforce.

9.2 We recommend assessing the impact of employment policies on health and inequalities in health (see also recommendation 1).

Housing and environment

10   We RECOMMEND policies which improve the availability of social housing for the less well off within a framework of environmental improvement, planning and design which takes into account social networks, and access to goods and services.

11   We RECOMMEND policies which improve housing provision and access to health care for both officially and unofficially homeless people.

12   We RECOMMEND policies which aim to improve the quality of housing. Specifically:

12.1 we recommend policies to improve insulation and heating systems in new and existing buildings in order to reduce further the prevalence of fuel poverty.

12.2 We recommend amending housing and licensing conditions and housing regulations on space and amenity to reduce accidents in the home, including measures to promote the installation of smoke detectors in existing homes.

13   We RECOMMEND the development of policies to reduce the fear of crime and violence, and to create a safe environment for people to live in.

Mobility, transport and pollution

14   We RECOMMEND the further development of a high quality public transport system which is integrated with other forms of transport and is affordable to the user.

15   We RECOMMEND further measures to encourage walking and cycling as forms of transport and to ensure the safe separation of pedestrians and cyclists from motor vehicles.

16   We RECOMMEND further steps to reduce the usage of motor cars to cut the mortality and morbidity associated with motor vehicle emissions.

17   We RECOMMEND further measures to reduce traffic speed, by environmental design and modification of roads, lower speed limits in built up areas, and stricter enforcement of speed limits.

18   We RECOMMEND concessionary fares should be available to pensioners and disadvantaged groups throughout the country, and that local schemes should emulate high quality schemes, such as those of London and the West Midlands.
     [. . .]

Mothers, children and families

21   We RECOMMEND policies which reduce poverty in families with children by promoting the material support of parents; by removing barriers to work for parents who wish to combine work with parenting; and by enabling those who wish to devote full-time to parenting to do so. Specifically:

21.1   we recommend an integrated policy for the provision of affordable, high quality day care and pre-school education with extra resources for disadvantaged communities (see also: recommendation 5).

       We recommend further reductions in poverty in women of child-bearing age, expectant mothers, young children and older people should be made by increasing benefits in cash or in kind to them (recommendation 3.1).

       We recommend measures to increase the uptake of benefits in entitled groups (recommendation 3.3).

22   We RECOMMEND policies which improve the health and nutrition of women of child-bearing age and their children with priority given to the elimination of food poverty and the prevention and reduction of obesity. Specifically:

We recommend further reductions in poverty in women of child-bearing age, expectant mothers, young children and older people should be made by increasing benefits in cash or in kind to them (recommendation 3.1).

We recommend further measures to improve the nutrition provided at school, including: the promotion of school food policies; the development of budgeting and cooking skills; the preservation of free school meals entitlement; the provision of free school fruit; and the restriction of less healthy food (recommendation 7).

We recommend a comprehensive review of the Common Agricultural Policy (CAP)'s impact on health and inequalities in health (recommendation 19).

We recommend policies which will increase the availability and accessibility of foodstuffs to supply an adequate and affordable diet (recommendation 20).

22.1 We recommend policies which increase the prevalence of breastfeeding.

22.2 We recommend the fluoridation of the water supply.

22.3 We recommend the further development of programmes to help women to give up smoking before or during pregnancy, and which are focused on the less well off.

23 We RECOMMEND policies that promote the social and emotional support for parents and children. Specifically:

23.1 we recommend the further development of the role and capacity of health visitors to provide social and emotional support to expectant parents, and parents with young children.

23.2 We recommend local authorities identify and address the physical and psychological health needs of looked-after children.

[. . .]

The National Health Service

37 We RECOMMEND that providing equitable access to effective care in relation to need should be a governing principle of all policies in the NHS. Priority should be given to the achievement of equity in the planning, implementation and delivery of services at every level of the NHS. Specifically:

37.1 we recommend extending the focus of clinical governance to give equal prominence to equity of access to effective health care.

37.2 We recommend extending the remit of the National Institute for Clinical Excellence to include equity of access to effective health care.

37.3 We recommend developing the National Service Frameworks to address inequities in access to effective primary care.

37.4 We recommend that performance management in relation to the national performance management framework is focused on achieving more equitable access, provision and targeting of effective services in relation to need in both primary and hospital sectors.

37.5   We recommend that the Department of Health and NHS Executive set out their responsibilities for furthering the principle of equity of access to effective health and social care, and that health authorities, working with Primary Care Groups and providers on local clinical governance, agree priorities and objectives for reducing inequities in access to effective care. These should form part of the Health Improvement Programme.

38   We RECOMMEND giving priority to the achievement of a more equitable allocation of NHS resources. This will require adjustments to the ways in which resources are allocated and the speed with which resource allocation targets are met. Specifically:

38.1   we recommend reviewing the "pace of change" policy to enable health authorities that are furthest from their capitation targets to move more quickly to their actual target.

38.2   We recommend extending the principle of needs-based weighting to non-cash limited General Medical Services (GMS) resources. The size and effectiveness of deprivation payments in meeting the needs and improving the health outcomes amongst the most disadvantaged populations, including ethnic minorities should be assessed.

38.3   We recommend reviewing the size and effectiveness of the Hospital and Community Health Service (HCHS) formula and deprivation payments in influencing the health care outcomes of the most dis-advantaged populations, and to consider alternative methods of focus-ing resources for health promotion and public health care to reduce health inequalities.

38.4   We recommend establishing a review of the relationship of private practice to the NHS with particular reference to access to effective treatments, resource allocation and availability of staff.

39   We RECOMMEND Directors of Public Health, working on behalf of health and local authorities, produce an equity profile for the popul-ation they serve, and undertake a triennial audit of progress towards achieving objectives to reduce inequalities in health.

39.1   We recommend there should be a duty of partnership between the NHS Executive and regional government to ensure that effective local partnerships are established between health, local authorities and other agencies and that joint programmes to address health inequalities are in place and monitored.

We RECOMMEND that as part of health impact assessment, all policies likely to have a direct or indirect effect on health should be evaluated in terms of their impact on health inequalities, and should be formulated in such a way that by favouring the less well off they will, wherever possible, reduce such inequalities (recommendation 1).

References

1 Dahlgren G, Whitehead M. *Policies and strategies to promote social equity in health.* Stockholm: Institute of Futures Studies, 1991.

2 Whitehead M. Tackling inequalities: a review of policy initiatives. In: Benzeval M, Judge K, Whitehead M, eds. *Tackling inequalities in health: an agenda for action.* London: Kings Fund, 1995.

3 House of Commons. Parliamentary debate. Oral Answers. *Hansard* 1997; **295**: Column 1139–1140.

4 Kuh B, Ben-Shlomo Y, eds. *A life course approach to chronic disease epidemiology.* Oxford: Oxford University Press, 1997.

5 Barker D. *Mothers, babies and health in later life.* Edinburgh: Churchill Livingstone, 1998.

Part III

Professionalisation and health

Introduction

Health and health care are dominated by medicine and the professionalisation of health is the focus for the selection of readings in the third section of the Reader.

Professionalisation has been seen by Freidson (Reading 17) to lend authority to a medical view and understanding of health and illness at the expense of lay views. The conflict between the perspectives of doctor and patient is seen to involve the submission of lay concerns about illness to a technical and scientific model of disease. The medical profession has been able to achieve this due to its ability, because of its professional status, to manage its own affairs 'protected from lay interference'. Autonomous and self-directing, and supported by the power of the state, the medical profession is able to 're-create the layman's world', defining and constructing illness in terms of its scientific and technical knowledge base. In this sense, Freidson emphasises that illness is 'socially defined', that it is a social product of the doctor–patient relationship rather than a feature of the patient's 'organic state'. Medicine's ability to dominate lay views does not involve a process of forcefully imposing its views on those of the lay person but instead requires the active co-operation of the layman in accepting the profession's right to authority in health matters. This co-operation is achieved in the process of interaction which occurs in the encounter between doctor and patient. As such, *both* (medical) professional and lay persons are active in contributing 'to the process of constructing the social reality of illness'. In the extract printed here, Freidson focuses on the increasing application of 'medical labels' in the control of social deviance. The reinterpretation of deviance as illness leads to 'the strengthening of a professionalised control institution' in which illness is defined as 'something bad' and medicine assumes the role of 'moral entrepreneur'.

Its scientific and professional status has enabled medicine to extend its authority and influence into new and expanding areas of jurisdiction. This process of 'medicalisation' has not, however, been seen to necessarily enhance health. This view is exemplified by Illich's extreme condemnation of medicalisation for its role in amplifying, rather than eradicating, illness. According to Illich (1976), medicine has done more harm than good insofar as its most far-reaching effects have been to create new health problems where none existed before and to disempower individuals by making us socially and culturally dependent upon medical expertise to solve our problems for us. Illich referred to this capacity of medicine to manufacture illness and dependency as 'iatrogenesis'.

Whatever the dangers of the professionalisation of health, the significance of the professions, and hence of medicine, to the maintenance of social order is evident from the role that 'expertise' has been increasingly called upon to fulfil in the governing of populations in the modern era. The transformation of professions in their relations to the state is explored in Johnson's discussion of 'Govermentality and the institutionalization of expertise' (Reading 18). Drawing on a range of work on professionalisation, and on Michel Foucault's notion of 'governmentality' (Foucault 1979), Johnson challenges interpretations of professionalisation which both view the state and the professions as distinct 'subjects', and their historical relationship as the gradual emergence of professional 'autonomy' from state 'intervention'. Instead, Johnson argues that the 'institutionalization of expertise in the form of the professions' has been central to the *establishing* of modern forms of government. In this sense the professions should not be viewed as an effect or outcome of the actions of the state but are instead to be seen as *part* of the state itself: 'The establishment of the jurisdiction of professions like medicine, psychiatry, law and accountancy, were all consequent on problems of government and, as such, were, from the beginning of the nineteenth century at least, the product of government programmes and policies. Far from emerging autonomously in a period of separation between state and society, the professions were part of the process of state formation' (Johnson 1995: 11).

That medicine fulfils a significant role as a mechanism of social control has long been recognised by medical sociologists. Talcott Parsons' classic formulation of the 'sick role' and analysis of the gate-keeping role of medicine in sanctioning socially legitimate sickness (Parsons 1951, 1978) represents an approach which sees in medicine's social role the exercise of expertise in the interests of all. For Parsons, medicine controls the potential social deviance of sickness by providing a legitimate 'sick role' to those prepared to exercise their illness in a socially approved fashion; that is, seeking to get well by consulting a medical practitioner and complying with prescribed treatment. This optimistic reading of the functioning of medicine has not gone unchallenged. Thus sociologists who emphasise links between medicine and the wider 'political economy', for instance, are led to very different conclusions regarding the social control effects of medical theory and practice. Vincente Navarro, for example, argues that a key function of medicine is to maintain and reproduce exploitative class relations through the interpretation and treatment of disease in terms of individual aetiology rather than as social phenomena (Navarro 1976).

In diverting attention away from the social origins of disease and illness medicine can both locate responsibility for illness in the sick themselves and support technologies which seek to identify potentially health damaging characteristics in healthy individuals. To this end medicine is increasingly being called upon to 'police' health, a development which Armstrong describes in accounting for the 'rise of surveillance medicine' (Reading 19). 'Surveillance medicine' is identified by Armstrong as emerging in the twentieth century as an alternative model to that of hospital-based biomedicine. Whilst biomedicine continues as the dominant model of medicine, focusing on the site of disease and intervention in the individual patient's body, surveillance medicine operates with a different focus which 'blurs the distinction between health and illness', namely the 'observation of seemingly healthy populations' for evidence of risks which may predict deteriorating health and the development of disease in the individual. The 'medical gaze' shifts from the body of the individual patient to the 'spaces between bodies' in the community. Surveillance medicine is seen to 'target everyone' and to encourage a strategy of self-surveillance in which each and every individual polices him/herself and remains vigilant against unchecked risk factors supported by discourses of 'lifestyle management' and 'health promotion'.

A significant component of medical surveillance has been the expansion and refinement of 'diagnostic testing' or 'screening'. The role of 'screening' in securing social regulation is explored in an extract from Lupton's critique of the 'imperative of health' (Reading 20), in which diagnostic testing is identified as a central technology of 'risk discourse' and which rational and socially responsible individuals are expected to utilise as part of their 'management of self'. Lupton draws our attention to the fact that screening is 'socially contextualized', emphasising that far from being the objective and value-free medical test for disease which public health and health promotion discourse says that it is, 'screening' is a 'social' rather than a 'technical' event, relying upon 'the social context of both doctor and patient' and with diagnosis involving an *interpretation* of the test results 'using subjective criteria'. Research into participation in medical tests reveals important differences in medical and lay understandings of the experience of the test and suggests that individuals seek tests for many different reasons, a conclusion at odds with the 'official' (medical) 'interpretation of the process'.

At the same time as medicine has been able to dominate the health field, significant challenges to 'medical hegemony' have been developing during the last thirty years or so. These are set to grow in pace as we move into the twenty-first century. The section ends with readings that illustrate three important dimensions of these challenges to the 'medical model'.

The 'public health' challenge to medicine questions the effectiveness of medical interventions in securing improvements in the population's health, suggesting that improved mortality and morbidity are the outcome of wider public health measures rather than of the intervention of medical science. This approach is illustrated here by an abridged extract (Reading 21) taken from the concluding chapter of Thomas McKeown's seminal *The Modern Rise of Population*, which challenged the long-established view that medical advances accounted for the large reductions in mortality from infectious disease and consequent growth in population size witnessed since the eighteenth century. Instead, McKeown locates the explanation first in improved nutrition resulting from the availability of greater food supplies made possible by agricultural advances, and second in the advances in hygiene which resulted in improvement in the quality of the environment through the public health measures of the late nineteenth century. In short, McKeown concludes that medical interventions have been far from crucial in improving the health of the population: 'the health of man is determined essentially by his behaviour, his food and the nature of the world around him, and is only marginally influenced by personal medical care'.

The 'managerial' challenge to medicine has its roots in government's desire to make health services more efficient, effective and economical. Such political goals impact on the traditional autonomy and control of resources which the medical profession has enjoyed and upon which its authority has largely been based. In his discussion of the 'managerial challenge to medical dominance' (Reading 22), Hunter raises the important question of how the medical profession may attempt to preserve and even extend its power and influence over health policy and practice in the face of 'managerialism'. Historically, the medical profession has retained its independence from the NHS, preserving a 'tribalistic mode of operating' rather than developing a 'corporate or collaborative one'. The pressure on the profession to embrace corporatism was intensified with the NHS reforms of the early 1990s. However, Hunter is not convinced that the ascendancy of managerialism seriously challenges medical dominance, for the reforms also offered doctors managerial opportunities (for example, clinical directors posts) which the profession could use to protect its power and authority. Indeed, the management agenda in the field of health is likely to remain 'medically defined': 'If a doctor is challenged to behave like his or her more efficient colleagues, the criteria of judgement are best *medical* practice and not *management* practice'. The outcome of the political and managerial challenge to medical dominance is therefore an open one, and particularly so if the medical profession is able to continue to attract widespread public support despite a recent series of high profile medical scandals including those associated with the Bristol Royal Infirmary and the trial and conviction of Harold Shipman.

In addition to those mounted by the 'new public health' movement and by 'managerialism', the medical profession faces a powerful and growing challenge from 'user' groups who reject its dismissive stance towards lay concerns and perspectives on health and illness. This challenge is represented here by an example (Reading 23) from work by the 'disability movement' which confronts and rejects the medical model of disability and advocates a 'social model' in its place. In the piece reprinted here, Colin Barnes focuses on a significant component of medicine's perspective on disability, namely its assumptions on how disability should be studied and what sort of knowledge should be produced. The medical model of disability supports and reproduces 'scientific' accounts in which the 'objectivity' and 'value neutrality' of the researcher are regarded as essential. Barnes rejects this view of research and of the role of the researcher in it, illustrating that whilst researchers might claim 'independence', their perspectives and research projects are heavily constrained by both a particular view of what counts as legitimate knowledge and by research and funding agendas which ultimately dictate what will and will not be researched and in what way it will be researched. Barnes argues that such 'independence' is not what the disability movement needs. Rather it requires 'commitment', 'engagement' and 'solidarity' from researchers as part of its overturning of the medical model of disability to reveal the social oppression of the disabled which this model and claims to independence in research mask.

References

Foucault, M. (1979) 'On governmentality', *Ideology and Consciousness* 6: 5–22.

Illich, I. (1976 [1990]) *Limits to Medicine. Medical Nemesis: The Expropriation of Health*, Harmondsworth: Penguin.

Johnson, T., Larkin, G. and Saks, M. (eds) (1995) *Health Professions and the State in Europe*, London: Routledge.

Navarro, V. (1976) *Medicine Under Capitalism*, New York: Prodist.

Parsons, T. (1951) *The Social System*, New York: The Free Press.

—— (1978) 'The sick role and the role of the physician reconsidered', in *Action Theory and the Human Condition*, New York: The Free Press, pp. 17–34.

17   The profession of medicine*

Eliot Freidson

The increasing emphasis on the label of illness, then, has been at the expense of the labels of both crime and sin and has been narrowing the limits if not weakening the jurisdiction of the traditional control institutions of religion and law. Indeed, my own suspicion is that the jurisdiction of the other institutions has been weakened absolutely because the thrust of the expansion of the application of medical labels has been toward addressing (and controlling) the *serious* forms of deviance, leaving to the other institutions a residue of essentially trivial or narrowly technical offenses.

The medical mode of response to deviance is thus being applied to more and more behavior in our society, much of which has been responded to in quite different ways in the past. In our day, what has been called crime, lunacy, degeneracy, sin, and even poverty in the past is now being called illness, and social policy has been moving toward adopting a perspective appropriate to the imputation of illness. Chains have been struck off and everywhere health professionalism has been raised to legitimate the claim that the proper management of deviance is "treatment" in the hands of a responsible and skilled profession. The labels of sin and crime being removed, what is done to the deviant is likely to be said to be done for his own good, done to help him rather than punish him, even though the treatment itself may constitute a deprivation under ordinary circumstances. His own opinions about his treatment are discounted because he is said to be a layman who lacks the special knowledge and detachment that would qualify him to have his voice heard.

This movement to reinterpret human deviance as illness has its roots in humanitarianism. As Wootton noted,

> Without question, therefore, in the contemporary attitude towards anti-social behavior, psychiatry and humanitarianism have marched hand in hand. Just because it is so much in keeping with the mental atmosphere of a scientifically-minded age, the medical treatment of social deviants has

*This is an extract from Freidson, E. (1970) *Profession of Medicine: A Study of the Sociology of Applied Knowledge*, University of Chicago Press, 1988 edition, pp. 249–55.

been a most powerful, perhaps even the most powerful, reinforcement of humanitarian impulses; for today the prestige of humane proposals is immensely enhanced if these are expressed in the idiom of medical science.[1]

The consequence of the movement, however, is the strengthening of a professionalized control institution that, in the name of the individual's good and of technical expertise, can remove from laymen the right to evaluate their own behavior and the behavior of their fellows – a fundamental right that is evidenced in a hard-won fight to interpret the Scriptures oneself, without regard to dogmatic authority, in religion and, the right to be judged by one's peers, in law.[2] The work of Thomas S. Szasz may be cited as a major effort to dissect the character of this newly emergent problem of the relationship of institutionalized expertise to the individual right of equality and self-determination.[3]

In evaluating the character of these developments, it is very important to separate demonstrable scientific achievement from the status of the occupation involved and the success it has had in establishing its jurisdiction. The jurisdiction that medicine has established extends far wider than its demonstrable capacity to "cure". Nonetheless, success at gaining general acceptance of the use of "illness" to label a disapproved form of behavior carries with it the assumption that the behavior is properly managed only by physicians. Similarly, the fact that physicians are willing to manage or deal with a problematic form of behavior leads to the illogical conclusion that the behavior must be an illness. For example, the "drunkard" is relabeled an "alcoholic", and "alcoholism" becomes a disease that should be treated by a physician rather than by the courts or the church. Such jurisdiction is established even though knowledge of etiology and a predictably successful method of treatment is as absent in medicine as it is in religion or law.[4] Thus, the medical profession has first claim to jurisdiction over the label of illness and anything to which it may be attached, irrespective of its capacity to deal with it effectively. In such a fashion do we see that the rise to social prominence of a social value such as health is inseparable from the rise of a vehicle for the value – an organized body of workers who claim jurisdiction over the value. Once official justification is gained, the profession is then prone to create its own specialized notions of what it is that shall be called illness. While medicine is hardly independent of the society in which it exists, by becoming a vehicle for society's values it comes to play a major role in the forming and shaping of the social meanings inbued with such value. What is the thrust of that role?

The physician as a moral entrepreneur

Clearly, neither medicine nor the physician may be characterized as passive. As a consulting rather than scholarly or scientific profession, medicine is committed to treatment rather than merely defining and studying man's ills. It has a mission of active intervention guided by what, in whatever time and place it exists, it believes to be ill in the world. Furthermore, it is active in seeking out illness. The profession does treat the illnesses layman take to it, but it also seeks to discover illness of which laymen may not even be aware. One of the greatest ambitions of the physicians is to discover and describe a 'new' disease or syndrome and to be immortalized by having his name used to identify the disease. Medicine, then, is oriented to seeking out and finding illness, which is to say that it seeks to create social meanings of illness where that meaning or interpretation was lacking before. And insofar as illness is defined as something bad – to be eradicated or contained – medicine plays the role of what Becker called the 'moral entrepreneur'.[5] Medical activity leads to the creation of new rules defining deviance; medical practice seeks to enforce those rules by attracting and treating the newly defined deviant sick.

At first thought it may seem peculiar to include the medical man with bluenoses, reformers, and others who are more obviously moral entrepreneurs. The physician's job is not generally seen to be moral; he is supposed to treat illness without judging. There is, however, an irreducible moral judgment in the designation of illness as such, a judgment the character of which is frequently overlooked because of the virtually universal consensus that exists about the undesirability of much of what is labeled illness. Cancer is so obviously undesirable to everyone that its status as an illness seems objective and self-evident rather than what it is – a social valuation on which most people happen to agree. Even recognizing this, however, it must be observed that the word "illness" is often used explicitly for the purpose of avoiding moral condemnation, for the humanitarian seeks to have it adopted in order that people will not be inclined to punish a deviant. By labeling something like alcoholism an "illness" and declaring an appallingly filthy derelict to be sick, the intention is to avoid moral condemnation.

However, while the label of illness does seem to function to discourage punitive reactions, it does not discourage condemnatory reactions. The "illness" is condemned rather than the person, but it is condemned nonetheless. The person is treated with sympathy rather than punishment, but he is expected to rid himself of the condemned attribute or behavior. Thus, while (ideally) the person may not be judged, his "disease" certainly is judged and his "disease" is part of him. Moral neutrality exists only when a person is *allowed* to be or do what he will, without remark or question. Positive moral approval, of course, exists where a person is *urged* to be what he may not wish to be. Clearly, the physician neither approves of disease nor is neutral to it. When he claims alcoholism is a disease, he is as much a moral entrepreneur as a fundamentalist who claims it is a sin. His mission is to impute social and therefore moral meaning to physical and other signs that are, but for such meaning, fit only for the licking and biting by which animals treat themselves.

However, there is a division of labor in such moral entrepreneurship in medicine. The everyday practitioner's task is to assign a medical label to symptoms that laymen have already singled out as undesirable. Clearly, on occasion the practitioner is a true entrepreneur when he finds illness of which the layman is unaware, but essentially his task is modest and unassuming. The major moral entrepreneurs in medicine are those seeking to influence public opinion and political policy, and of these there seem to be three kinds. There are, first, the public spokesmen for the organized profession or its specialties. They seek to alert the public to the important dangers of a given disease or of the virtues of a given kind of health – dental, mental, or otherwise. Their activities tend to be fairly sober and technical appeals for the public to undertake preventive health practices, including seeing their physicians. Second, there are the major moral entrepreneurs of medicine itself, some of whom may be individual practitioners whose avocation is crusading in health matters, but most of whom are not full-time practitioners at all; instead, they are associated with organized community health institutions like hospitals, clinics, medical schools, and health departments. These are the technical advisers who are interviewed most commonly by the public press on issues of health policy and who are called to give testimony before legislative bodies. The thrust of their activity is toward political power to implement measures designed to improve what they see to be the public health. In association with representatives of organized medical interests, and reinforced by interested lay bodies, they have also been responsible for most of the legislation that has, in the name of humanitarianism, attempted to remove such ills as alcoholism, drug addiction, mental illness, and mental deficiency from the jurisdiction of the courts and to place them under the jurisdiction of the health professions.

Finally may be mentioned the special lay interest groups, sometimes led by physicians but always including at least one prominent physician, which crusades each against the menace of its own specially chosen disease, impairment, or presumably disease-inducing agent.[6] Here, untrammeled by professional dignity, are the most flamboyant moral entrepreneurs in health, each concerned with arousing the public to give it the attention and resources that can only be gained at the expense of the other, each trying to create in the public mind profound pity and horror at its own specially chosen human failing. Some groups are concerned with establishing the application of the label of illness to conditions not considered illness before (as in the case of alcoholism), others with removing the stigma of some diseases (like leprosy) by changing their labels (to Hansen's disease), and others with redefining an illness (like epilepsy) so that it moves in the public mind from the category of chronic, serious, or incurable to minor or at least curable or controllable.

With the possible exception of the everyday practitioner, who spends most of his working time on routine and minor ailments and who has occasion to relieve his patients of worry (and relieve himself of patients worrying at him) by deprecating their symptoms and stressing their health, most of the activities of the active moral entrepreneurs of health are permeated by the tendency to see more illness everywhere around and to see the environment as being more dangerous to health than does the layman.[7] Impatient of available statistics based on the number of cases actually diagnosed and reported by everyday practitioners, they are prone to emphasize the seriousness of the health problem preoccupying them by estimating the cases presently undiagnosed and therefore untreated. Their estimates, furthermore, are likely to be based on a broader definition of the illness or impairment than the public uses – seeing "blindness" where the layman sees extremely bad vision,[8] "mental illness" where the layman sees "nervousness" or "problems", and "alcoholism" where the layman sees "heavy drinking". In short, the moral entrepreneur in medical affairs is likely to see illness where the layman sees something other than illness, or sees merely individual variation within broad boundaries of the normal. And he is likely to see a serious problem where the layman sees a minor one. They are biased toward illness as such and toward creating secondary deviance – sick roles – where before there was but primary deviance.

Notes

1 Barbara Wootton, *Social Science and Social Pathology* (London: George Allen and Unwin, 1959), p. 206.
2 "Thus the medicalization of deviance results in the political castration of the deviant." Jesse R. Pitts, "Social Control: The Concept," *International Encyclopedia of the Social Sciences* (New York: The Macmillan Company and The Free Press, 1968), Vol. XIV, p. 391.
3 Thomas S. Szasz, *Law, Liberty and Psychiatry* (New York: The Macmillan Co., 1963).
4 The desire to do away with the punitive treatment of alcoholics leads even so sophisticated a student as Jellinek to the curious tactic of noting that while no one has untangled the facts sufficiently to know the cause or cure of "alcoholism" (if it is a single entity rather than many separate ones, each with a different "cause"), nonetheless it is a disease. What is a disease? "*A disease is what the medical profession recognizes as such.*" That is, we do not know what the causes are, but because physicians call it a disease, it must therefore be something caused by natural forces over which the deviant has no control! See E. M. Jellinek, *The Disease Concept of Alcoholism* (New Haven: Hillhouse Press, 1960), p. 12. And see Thomas S. Szasz, "Alcoholism: a Socio-Ethical Perspective," *Washburn Law Journal,* VI (1667), 255–268.
5 See Howard S. Becker, *Outsiders* (New York: The Free Press of Glencoe, 1963), pp. 147–163.
6 See the provocative discussion in Joseph R. Gusfield, *Symbolic Crusade, Status Politics and the American Temperance Movement* (Urbana: University of Illinois Press, 1966). And see Joseph R. Gusfield, "Moral Passage: The Symbolic Process in Public Designations of Deviance," *Social Problems,* XV (1967), 175–188.
7 It is in the light of these comments that it may be profitable to evaluate the finding that "underreporting of symptoms [by laymen] is a more prevalent problem than overreporting," in S. V. Kasl and Sidney Cobb, "Health Behavior, Illness Behavior and Sick Role Behavior," *Archives of Environmental Health,* XII (1966), 256.
8 For an enlightening analysis of blindness see Robert A. Scott, *The Making of Blind Men* (New York: Russell Sage Foundation, 1969).

18 Governmentality and the institutionalization of expertise*

Terry Johnson

Larson and Foucault: expertise and governmentality

In order to extricate ourselves from the distorting consequences of the state/profession dualism, we must first rid our thinking of the concept of the state as a preconstituted, calculating subject. We must also develop a more balanced view of both the state and the professions as the structured outcomes of political objectives and governmental programmes rather than seeing them as either the constraining environments of action or the preconstituted agents of action. We can move further in this direction by considering the significance for our argument of the work of sociologists Larson (1977) and Abbott (1988), both of whom emphasize the processual nature of the social construction of expertise. Like Freidson, Larson and Abbott offer relatively sophisticated analyses of the professions, the former viewing professionalization as primarily the construction of a market in professional commodities or services; the latter identifying professionalism as a system of competitive occupational relations centring on jurisdictional claims and disputes.

For Larson, the market in professional services, as it emerged in the nineteenth century, depended on the production of a distinctive commodity. It being in the nature of a professional commodity to be inextricably 'bound to the person and personality of the producer' (Larson 1977: 14), it follows that the creation of a distinctive service requires the prior training, socialization and public establishment of a recognizable producer. Here, like Foucault, Larson links the emergence of the techniques and procedures of expertise to the reproduction of trained subjects. However, Foucault's analysis takes a different course to that of Larson, focusing on the normalization of the self-regulating, subject-client (the client, patient), rather than the subject-producer (the expert, professional). Foucault is interested in the general process of governmentality; its disciplines and its objects. Larson is concerned with the construction and institutionalization of expertise; one strand of governmentality.

*This is an extract from a chapter first published in Johnson, T., Larkin, G., and Saks, M. (eds) (1995) *Health Professions and the State in Europe*, Routledge, pp. 7–24.

For Larson the creation of an established market in professional commodities required that 'stabled criteria of evaluation' were fixed in the minds
of consumer-clients. This process of commodity standardization was associated with the elimination of alternative criteria of evaluation and, therefore, of
alternative practitioners. Larson, in keeping with other sociologists, regards
the elimination of 'quacks' as centrally significant to the monopolization of
expertise associated with professionalization. But Foucault once again shifts
our attention to the governing process and its dependence on the establishment of uniform definitions of reality. Larson, by stressing the professional
drive towards practice monopoly, tends to underplay the importance for the
governing process of the establishment of universally recognized definitions of
social reality. As Miller and Rose point out, such definitions render

> aspects of existence thinkable and calculable, and amenable to deliberate
> and planful initiatives; a complex intellectual labour involving not only
> the invention of new forms of thought, but also the invention of novel
> procedures of documentation, computation and evaluation.
>
> (1990: 3)

It is in such a context that the existence of competing forms of expertise not
only undermines the professionalizing strategies of occupations, but also
reduces the coherence of government programmes.

Larson (1977): 14–18) comes close to Foucault when she suggests that in
the development of the modern professions commodity standardization was
but one aspect of a wider process of 'ideological persuasion', itself part of a
newly emerging symbolic universe. According to Larson (1977: 15), the state,
'the supreme legitimising and enforcing institution', was fundamental to
securing the conditions of professionalization. The 'conquest of official
privilege' was essential in constructing that public 'monopoly of credibility'
(Larson 1977: 17) which today remains central to the creation of a professional commodity. However favoured an occupation might be in the
division of labour, the creation of a realm of cognitive exclusiveness as part of
a successful project of market control depended on the supporting role of the
state. Larson quotes Polanyi (1957) approvingly:

> the road to the free market was opened and kept open by an enormous
> increase in continuous, centrally organized and controlled intervention-
> ism . . . There was nothing natural about laissez-faire . . . laissez-faire itself
> was enforced by the state.
>
> (1977: 53)

State-backed monopoly was, Larson claims, the mechanism through which
professions 'protected themselves against the undue interference of the state'
(1977: 53).

In seeking to explain the rise of the professions, then, Larson comes to
much the same conclusion as Freidson; that it is state intervention or 'shelter'

that secures professional autonomy – the paradox is restated. As with Freidson, the value of Larson's analysis lies in the fact that she also refuses to sit secure on one or other side of the dualist see-saw of state intervention and professional autonomy. In Larson's analysis autonomy depends on intervention, not on this occasion because autonomy and intervention refer to two different objects (that is, technical evaluation as against socio-economic organization) but because intervention is construed as a class strategy in which state intervention favours the bourgeoisie – in this case the professional segment of the bourgeoisie: 'Indeed, reliance upon the state was not merely a pattern borrowed by the nineteenth-century professions from the medieval guilds, but also the means by which the ascending bourgeoisie had advanced toward a self-regulating market' (Larson 1977: 53). There is in Larson's account, then, no necessity for autonomy to be built into the technicality of expertise. Rather, professional autonomy is seen as an historical emergent; part of the processes of class and state formation. By stressing the historical specificity of professionalization and its links to state and class formation Larson draws a little closer to Foucauldian analysis. However, her argument is of particular value when she introduces Gramscian theory to suggest that: 'Intellectuals are obviously of strategic importance for the ruling class, whose power cannot rest on coercion alone but needs to capture the moral and intellectual direction of society as a whole.' (Larson 1977: xiv).

This 'organic' tie to a rising class identifies professionals as potentially privileged bodies of experts, officially entrusted with the task of defining a sector or reality in a way that underpins established or emergent power; whether that be conceived of as state power or class power. This reference to Gramsci identifies an important aspect of the profession/state complex that is often noted, but only emerges as a systematic concern in Foucauldian analysis. Namely, the fact that expertise not only functions as a system of legitimation, but is institutionalized as part of the governing and legitimating processes.

While both Larson and Freidson emphasize that professional expertise has been dependent on governments for recognition, licence and legitimation, they are not so systematically emphatic that the professions, in constructing an officially recognized realm of social reality, are also a significant source of the growing capacity for governing, expressed by Foucault in the concept of governmentality. Foucault's argument deepens our understanding of these interdependencies of class, state and professions, by focusing on what Larson refers to as the 'new symbolic universe' associated with the rise of the professions. This emergent pattern of cognitive and normative changes – the 'great transformation' – not only generated the popular legitimations underpinning liberal, democratic government, but also induced what Stanley Cohen (1985), after Foucault, has called a profound shift in the 'master patterns of social control'. This shift included the construction of new deviancy control systems, the institutional expressions of which were the 'austere' and 'rational' bureaucratic organizations created for the classification and segregation of the poor, the criminal, the mad, the sick and the young. It is from Foucault that we derive the view that government and the professions were inextricably fused in this 'transformation' of the 'strategies and technologies' of power. Both were the progenitors and, in part, the beneficiaries of this complex network of interrelated social realities which constituted the various emergent realms of expertise and rendered them governable.

If at this stage of the argument we continue to insist on the dualism, state/profession, the word juggling becomes extreme. For we are forced to conclude not only that the independence of the professions depends on the interventions of the state, but that the state is dependent on the independence of the professions in securing the capacity to govern as well as legitimating its governance. The obvious implication of all this is to suggest that we must develop ways of talking about state and profession that conceive of the relationship not as a struggle for autonomy or control but as the interplay of integrally related structures, evolving as the combined product of occupational strategies, governmental policies and shifts in public opinion.

Abbott and Foucault: realms of expertise and governmentality

This conclusion brings us to Abbott's *The System of Professions*, a recent and fruitful sociological perspective, worth considering here insofar as it insists that the 'real, the determining history of the professions' (1988: 2) lies in competitive struggles between occupations for jurisdiction over realms of expertise. According to Abbott, experts are continuously engaged in making claims and counter-claims for jurisdiction over existing, emergent and vacant areas of expertise. These are the very same realms of expertise that Foucault identifies as enabling and empowering governmentality. In short, far from avoiding politics by way of the adoption of a neutral stance or the establishment of autonomy, professionals are always, in their jurisdictional competitions, intimately involved in politics; the politics of governmentality.

The value of Abbott's approach for us lies not so much in his focus on the professions as a 'system' of such competitive relationships, but in the claim that the established professions – institutionalized expertise – are emergent from such a competitive, political process. Abbott advances beyond the conventional sociological literature, then, in focusing *not* on the precon-stituted professional subject seeking autonomy, but on the processes through which occupations constitute and reproduce themselves, relative to others, as professions.

The degree to which this approach, by focusing on the political process of jurisdictional claims, suggests a dismemberment of the intervention/ autonomy couple is once again undermined by Abbott's insistence on the duality of state and profession. For example, Abbott's model suggests that the system of competitive interdependencies that generates a profession has its origins in negotiated jurisdictions in the workplace; jurisdictions which are thereafter generalized through the establishment of such claims first in the arena of public opinion and then in the legal order (Abbott 1988: 59–61);

this last linking nicely with the problematic of governmentality. In Abbott's analysis, however, it is only at the point at which the legal order is brought into play that the state emerges, as a preconstituted, calculating subject.

The state is conceived largely as an audience for professional claims. In other words the state is an environmental factor in the system of professions; an external agent made up of the legislature, the courts and the administrative or planning structure (Abbott 1988: 63–3). The typical sequence of events in the establishment of a professional jurisdiction involves the success of an occupation in workplace negotiations, followed by an accepted claim in the public arena of opinion, and only then a 'crowning' of these earlier successes by way of legal recognition.

The initial problem that arises for such an analysis is that it is difficult to sustain the validity of this sequence of events for the development of the professions in any country other than the United States. However, according to Abbott, while the sequence is crucial in establishing professional claims in the United States, in a number of continental European countries the state rather than public opinion has, untypically, constituted the primary audience for jurisdictional claims. In these cases, he argues, public opinion coalesces with the administration and the legal order to constitute the 'common opinion of state officials' (Abbott 1988: 60).

By identifying the state in terms of its organizational locations (the courts, legislature, administration) and its interventionist capacity (Abbott 1988: 163), and by separating both of these from the arena of public opinion, Abbott leaves himself with no effective means of incorporating the wider politics of state formation into his jurisdictional analysis, despite the fact that his work leads one in that very direction. In short, the reactive state (pro-active in the case of France (Abbott 1988: 158–62) is divorced from the public arena, while work-site negotiations are cut off from public and national processes of claim and counter-claim. Abbott's concept of 'audiences' for professional claims cuts across the field of political struggles, so submerging their effects.

For Foucault the concept of governmentality incorporates the politics of expertise, which are, at one and the same time, made up of Abbott's occupational competition over jurisdictions, the politics of policy formation and the politics of state formation. If we recognize that both public opinion and government constitute, along with the experts themselves, agents in a political process, then we must reject the implication in Abbott's analysis that governments are typically latecomers on the scene, uninvolved in the formation of public opinion or the work-site formation of occupational jurisdictions.

In centring his analysis on the interplay of jurisdictional claims, Abbott focuses on the professions as an emergent set of properties arising out of occupational strategies. The state remains conceptualized as a preconstituted, reactive agent rather than itself an emergent property of the system. Once we include governments and administrators as participating equally with the experts in Abbott's complex of jurisdictional claims, then we also describe part of the process that Foucault calls governmentality. Once we follow Foucault in conceptualizing the state as the outcome of these interrelations, then we can begin to look at the issues associated with the institutionalization of expertise in a manner quite other than that imposed on us by the state intervention/ professional autonomy couple.

One result of such a reconceptualization will be the recognition that the 'neutrality' of professional expertise, where it exists, is itself an outcome of a political process rather than the product of some inherent essence, such as esoteric knowledge. Once we see institutionalized expertise as an aspect of governmentality then it is possible to recognize that professionalization begins not only with the adoption of occupational strategies, but also with the formation of government programmes and objectives.

Starr and Immergut: the changing boundaries of politics

These issues can be elaborated further by way of a consideration of yet another recent contribution to the sociology of the professions, the article by Starr and Immergut (1987) on 'Health care and the boundaries of politics'. Their thesis, relating to governmental health policies, effectively resituates Abbott's argument regarding the establishment of professional jurisdictions by focusing on politics as a sphere in which various interests, groups and individuals struggle over and 'seek to shape the uses of governmental power' (Starr and Immergut 1987: 222). This contribution brings us closer to the Foucauldian perspective insofar as governmentality is an attempt to specify the nature of government power in modern societies.

According to Starr and Immergut the general sphere of politics has the capacity to expand and contract. In periods of rapid social change, for example, arenas of decision-making once considered realms of neutral, objective fact may be reconstituted as politically contentious. That is to say, matters which Freidson might identify as of purely technical concern – to be resolved by recognized experts – erupt into 'political controversy'.

In Britain, we have recently experienced a number of such eruptions, largely as a result of the Thatcher government's policy initiatives of the 1980s; policies affecting a variety of professions including medicine, education, law and planning. As long ago as 1974 Sir Keith Joseph, the first Thatcherite Minister of Education, indicated what was to come when he made the following comments on planning and planners:

> It is not only that the pursuit of town planning aims intensifies land shortage, prolongs delays, increases devastation, imposes rigid lifeless solutions; it is not only that town planning makes the artificial shortages that lead to the fortunes that feed envy; it is not only that the ambitious system of town planning leads to long administrative delays with heavy concealed costs all round on top of the visible costs of a big bureaucracy;

it is not only that any system leading to such wide disparities of land values must offer a temptation to corruption; it is that town planners and architects are as fallible as the rest of us and the more power we give them the greater errors that will be made when they are wrong.

(quoted in Cherry 1982: 69)

Joseph's attack represented a rupture of the postwar political consensus which viewed professional town planning as one of the glories of the welfare state. His remarks also drew on an immense well of public disillusionment over urban town planning in particular (Dennis 1972), and a growing scepticism about the role of the professions in general.

The implications of Joseph's remarks did not emerge fully, however, until the third term of the Thatcher government, when the elements that made up the overall policy towards expert services began to fall into place – the Education Reform Bill, the Health Services White Paper, the Green Paper on Legal Services, the White Paper on the Reorganization of Broadcasting, and the Monopoly and Mergers Commission Reports on professional advertising. Together these events constituted an unprecedented shake-up in the jurisdictions and organization of expert services, with potential effects rivalling the privatizations of state-run industries.

The overall objectives of government policy also became increasingly clear. While the government was attempting to achieve a variety of specific policy goals relating to the provision of legal services, the stock market, the National Health Service, the universities and the schools, each of these cases also illustrated an overall policy commitment to cost effectiveness, accountability, competition and consumer choice. The common assumption behind each discrete reform was that the high and spiralling costs of expert services – some argued of professional privilege – were no longer acceptable.

A rapidly ageing population rendered the problem of cost particularly acute in the field of health care. The legal services were increasingly threatened by the pressure on legal aid, while in further and higher education the government's commitment to a policy of rapid expansion threatened a further cost explosion. The government's response to these compounded issues was the establishment of systems of monitoring, audit and appraisal as means of controlling costs. Whether applied by the professionals themselves or by external agencies these systems have, along with associated policies, the potential to redefine the boundaries between professional occupations, as well as the relations between professionals and their clients. In many cases it is too early to assess the full effects of such reforms, but it is clear that the boundaries defining expert jurisdictions and realms of neutrality are in process of transformation.

For example, the systems of financial and medical audit developed in respect of general practice and hospitals in the National Health Service have become hot political issues, centred on the competing criteria of 'cost' and 'care'. Cost criteria, it has been argued by the medical profession, are likely to

distort the clinical judgements of general practitioner budget-holders, particularly in respect of the elderly and the chronically ill, who would become a
drain on practice budgets funded in accordance with an undifferentiated per
capita rate. What were once accepted as technical matters best determined
within the confines of the general practitioner's consulting room have become
burning political issues. The point is that changing government objectives
have had the effect of shifting the boundaries between what was regarded as
contentious and what was accepted as neutral. To put it in another way, the
arenas of professional neutrality and autonomy are transformed, not as a
product of changing occupational strategies, as Abbott would have it; not as
an effect of technical change, as suggested by Freidson; but as a result of
changing government objectives and policies.

As government objectives alter, transforming the boundaries of politics, so
too do professional jurisdictions and the established powers and functions of
the state. The point is central to Foucault's view of governmentality:

> [Since] it is the tactics of the government which make possible the
> continual definition and redefinition of what is within the competence of
> the State and what is not, the public versus the private, and so on; thus
> the State can only be understood in its survival and its limits on the basis
> of the general tactics of governmentality.
>
> (Foucault 1979: 21)

The processes as described by Starr and Immergut are just these tactics of
governmentality. They are the policy-triggered politicizations and depoliticiz-
ations which constantly 'disturb established rights and powers' (Starr and
Immergut 1987: 222), including those of experts. A crucial aspect of what
they call the 'permanent structure' of the modern liberal state are the
boundaries which conventionally and legally demarcate distinctions between
the public and the private, between the technical and the political and, it
follows, between the professions and the state:

> [Professional] or administrative sphere in government, which they hold
> separate from politics. Indeed, the military, civil service, scientific agencies
> and public health services are generally not only thought but legally
> required to be divorced from politics in the restricted but important sense
> of being nonpartisan and professional.
>
> (Starr and Immergut 1987: 225)

The authors make it clear that the notion of boundary is, in their usage,
merely a spatial metaphor which lends 'an exaggerated fixity' to these
distinctions which are in reality 'ambiguous, multiple and overlapping' (Starr
and Immergut, 1987: 251) as well as being politically and intellectually contested. Nevertheless, it remains the case that in modern democracies such
boundaries are maintained even when, as observation shows, they are charac-

terized by continuous movement. In short, those outcomes of governmentality we call the state, including those bodies of experts and expertise that both make it up yet are differentiated from it, are always in process of *becoming*.

References

Abbott, A. (1988) *The System of Professions: An Essay on the Division of Expert Labor*, Chicago: University of Chicago Press.

Cherry, G. (1982) *The Politics of Town Planning*, London: Longman.

Cohen, S. (1985) *Visions of Social Control*, Cambridge: Polity Press.

Dennis, N (1972) *Public Participation and Planners' Blight*, London: Faber.

Foucault, M. (1979) 'On governmentality', *Ideology and Consciousness* 6: 5–22.

Larson, M. S. (1977) *The Rise of Professionalism: A Sociological Analysis*, Berkeley: University of California Press.

Miller, P. and Rose, N. (1990) 'Governing economic life', *Economy and Society* 19(1): 1–31.

Polanyi, K. (1957) *The Great Transformation*, Boston: Beacon Press.

Starr, P. and Immergut, E. (1987) 'Health care and the boundaries of politics', in C. S. Maier (ed.), *Changing Boundaries of the Political*, Cambridge: Cambridge University Press.

19 The rise of surveillance medicine*

David Armstrong

Problematisation of the normal

Hospital Medicine was only concerned with the ill patient in whom a lesion might be identified, but a cardinal feature of Surveillance Medicine is its targeting of everyone. Surveillance Medicine requires the dissolution of the distinct clinical categories of healthy and ill as it attempts to bring everyone within its network of visibility. Therefore one of the earliest expressions of Surveillance Medicine – and a vital precondition for its continuing proliferation – was the problematisation of the normal.

No doubt there were nineteenth century manifestations of the idea that a person – or more frequently, a population – hung precariously between health and illness (such as the attempts to control the health of prostitutes near military establishments with the Contagious Diseases Acts), but it was the child in the twentieth century that became the first target of the full deployment of the concept. The significance of the child was that it underwent growth and development: there was therefore a constant threat that proper stages might not be negotiated that in its turn justified close medical observation. The establishment and wide provision of antenatal care, birth notification, baby clinics, milk depots, infant welfare clinics, day nurseries, health visiting and nursery schools ensured that the early years of child development could be closely monitored (Armstrong 1983). For example, the School Medical (later Health) Service not only provided a traditional 'treatment' clinic, but also provided an 'inspection' clinic that screened all school children at varying times for both incipient and manifest disease, and enabled visits to children's homes by the school nurse to report on conditions and monitor progress (HMSO 1975).

In parallel with the intensive surveillance of the body of the infant during the early twentieth century, the new medical gaze also turned to focus on the unformed mind of the child. As with physical development, psychological growth was construed as inherently problematic, precariously normal. The

*This is an extract from Armstrong, D. 'The rise of surveillance medicine', *Sociology of Health & Illness*, vol. 17, no. 3, pp. 393–404, 1995.

initial solution was for psychological well-being to be monitored and its abnormal forms identified. (The contemporary work of Freud that located adult psychopathology in early childhood experience can be seen as part of this approach.) The nervous child, the delicate child, the eneuretic child, the neuropathic child, the maladjusted child, the difficult child, the neurotic child, the over-sensitive child, the unstable child and the solitary child, all emerged as a new way of seeing a potentially hazardous normal childhood (Armstrong 1983, Rose 1985, 1990).

If there is one image that captured the nature of the machinery of observation that surrounded the child in those early decades of the twentieth century, it might well be the height and weight growth chart. Such charts contain a series of gently curving lines, each one representing the growth trajectory of a population of children. Each line marked the 'normal' experience of a child who started his or her development at the beginning of the line. Thus, every child could be assigned a place on the chart and, with successive plots, given a personal trajectory. But the individual trajectory only existed in a context of general population trajectories: the child was unique yet uniqueness could only be read from a composition which summed the unique features of all children. A test of normal growth assumed the possibility of abnormal growth, yet how, from knowledge of other children's growth, could the boundaries of normality be identified? When was a single point on the growth and weight chart, to which the sick child was reduced, to be interpreted as abnormal? Abnormality was a relative phenomenon. A child was abnormal with reference to other children, and even then only by degrees. In effect, the growth charts were significant for distributing the body of the child in a field delineated not by the absolute categories of physiology and pathology, but by the characteristics of the normal population.

The socio-medical survey, first introduced during World War II to assess the perceived health status of the population, represented the recruitment to medicine of an efficient technical tool that both measured and reaffirmed the extensiveness of morbidity. The survey revealed the ubiquity of illness, that health was simply a precarious state. The post-war fascination with the weakening person–patient interface – such as in the notion of the clinical iceberg which revealed that most illness lay outside of health care provision (Last 1963), or of illness behaviour which showed that people experience symptoms most days of their lives yet very few were taken to the doctor (Mechanic and Volkart 1960) – was evidence that the patient was inseparable from the person because all persons were becoming patients.

The survey also demanded alternative ways of measuring illness that would encompass nuances of variation from some community-based idea of the normal. Hence the development of health profile questionnaires, subjective health measures, and other survey instruments with which to identify the proto-illness and its sub-clinical manifestations, and latterly the increasing importance of qualitative methodologies that best capture illness as an experience rather than as a lesion (Fitzpatrick *et al.* 1984).

The results of the socio-medical survey threw into relief the important distinction between the biomedical model's binary separation of health and disease, and the survey's continuous distribution of variables throughout the population. The survey classified bodies on a continuum: there were no inherent distinctions between a body at one end and one at the other, their only differences were the spaces that separated them. (Perhaps the celebrated debate between Pickering and Platt on whether blood pressure was bimodally or continuously distributed in the population was another manifestation of this disharmony between alternative ways of reading the nature of illness (Pickering 1962).) The referent external to the population under study, which had for almost two centuries governed the analysis of bodies, was replaced by the relative positions of all bodies. Surveillance Medicine fixed on these gaps between people to establish that everyone was normal yet no-one was truly healthy.

For a long time, in the past, death came in the shape of a black-cloaked figure to mark the end of life: such deaths were natural in as much as it was nature that came to reclaim her own. The advent of Hospital Medicine two hundred years ago transformed the natural death into the pathological one (Foucault 1973). Death did not come from outside life, but was contained within life from the moment of birth – or, more correctly, conception – as physiological and pathological processes battled for supremacy. (Though it took biomedicine nearly a century to abolish the designation of death from 'natural causes' (Smith 1979).) Since the 1960s the analysis of death has again shifted. Medical professionals are now encouraged to persuade the dying to speak the truth about their death to the listening ear (Armstrong 1987). The surveillance machinery is trained to hear the anxieties of the dying and through reflection normalise them: the natural death, the pathological death, and now the normal death.

Dissemination of intervention

The blurring of the distinction between health and illness, between the normal and the pathological, meant that health care intervention could no longer focus almost exclusively on the body of the patient in the hospital bed. Medical surveillance would have to leave the hospital and penetrate into the wider population.

The new 'social' diseases of the early twentieth century – tuberculosis, venereal disease, problems of childhood, the neuroses, etc. – were the initial targets for novel forms of health care, but the main expansion in the techniques of monitoring occurred after World War II when an emphasis on comprehensive health care, and primary and community care, underpinned the deployment of explicit surveillance services such as screening and health promotion. But these later radiations out into the community were prefigured by two important inter-war experiments in Britain and the United States that demonstrated the practicality of monitoring precarious normality in a whole population.

The British innovation was the Pioneer Health Centre at Peckham in south London (Pearse and Crocker 1943). The Centre offered ambulatory health care to local families that chose to register – but the care placed special emphasis on continuous observation. From the design of its buildings that permitted clear lines of sight to its social club that facilitated silent observation of patients' spontaneous activity, every development within the Peckham Centre was a conscious attempt to make visible the web of human relations. Perhaps the Peckham key summarises the dream of this new surveillance apparatus. The key and its accompanying locks were designed (though never fully installed) to give access to the building and its facilities for each individual of every enrolled family. But as well as giving freedom of access, the key enabled a precise record of all movement within the building. 'Suppose the scientist should wish to know what individuals are using the swimming bath or consuming milk, the records made by the use of the key give him this information' (Pearse and Crocker 1943:76–7).

Only 7 per cent of those attending the Peckham Centre were found to be truly healthy; and if everyone had pathology then everyone would need observing. An important mechanism for operationalising this insight was the introduction of extensive screening programmes in the decades following World War II. However, screening, whether individual, population, multi-phasic, or opportunistic, represented a bid by Hospital Medicine to reach out beyond its confines – with all its accompanying limitations. First, it was too focused on the body. It meant that screening still confronted the localised lesion (or, more commonly, proto-lesion) within the body and ignored the newly emerging mobile threats that were insinuated throughout the community, constantly reforming into new dangers. Second, techniques to screen the population have always had to confront points of resistance, particularly the unwillingness of many to participate in these new procedures. The solution to these difficulties had already begun to emerge earlier in the twentieth century with the development of a strategy that involved giving responsibility for surveillance to patients themselves. A strategy of health promotion could potentially circumvent the problems inherent in illness screening.

The process through which the older techniques of hygiene were trans-formed into the newer strategy of health promotion occurred over several decades during the twentieth century. But perhaps one of the earliest experiments that attempted the transition was the collaborative venture between the city of Fargo in North Dakota and the Commonwealth Fund in 1923. The nominal objective of the project was the incorporation of child health services into the permanent programme of the health department and public school system (Brown 1929) and an essential component of this plan was the introduction of health education in Fargo's schools, supervised by Maud Brown. Brown's campaign was, she wrote, 'an attempt to secure the instant adoption by every child of a completely adequate program of health behaviour' (Brown 1929:19).

Prior to 1923 the state had required that elements of personal hygiene he taught in Fargo's schools 'but there was no other deliberately planned link between the study of physical well-being and the realization of physical well-being'. The Commonwealth Fund project was a two pronged strategy. While the classroom was the focus for a systematic campaign of health behaviour, a periodic medical and dental examination both justified and monitored the educational intervention. In effect 'health teaching, health supervision and their effective coordination' were linked together. In Fargo 'health teaching departed from the hygiene textbook, and after a vitalizing change, found its way back to the textbook' (Brown 1929:19). From its insistence on four hours of physical exercises a day – two of them outdoors – to its concern with the mental maturation of the child, Fargo represented the realization of a new public health dream of surveillance in which everyone is brought into the vision of the benevolent eye of medicine through the medicalisation of everyday life.

After World War II this approach began to be deployed with more vigour in terms of a strategy of health promotion. Concerns with diet, exercise, stress, sex, etc., become the vehicles for encouraging the community to survey itself. The ultimate triumph of Surveillance Medicine would be its internalisation by all the population.

The tactics of Hospital Medicine have been those of exile and enclosure. The lesion marked out those who were different in a great binary system of illness and health, and processed them (in the hospital) in an attempt to rejoin them to the healthy. The tactics of the new Surveillance Medicine, on the other hand, have been pathologisation and vigilance. The techniques of health promotion recognise that health no longer exists in a strict binary relationship to illness, rather health and illness belong to an ordinal scale in which the healthy can become healthier, and health can co-exist with illness; there is now nothing incongruous in having cancer yet believing oneself to be essentially healthy (Kagawa-Singer 1993). But such a trajectory towards the healthy state can only be achieved if the whole population comes within the purview of surveillance: a world in which everything is normal and at the same time precariously abnormal, and in which a future that can be transformed remains a constant possibility.

Spatialisation of risk factors

The extension of a medical eye over all the population is the outward manifestation of the new framework of Surveillance Medicine. But more fundamentally there is a concomitant shift in the primary spatialisation of illness as the relationship between symptom, sign and illness are reconfigured. From a linkage based on surface and depth, all become components in a more general arrangement of predictive factors.

A symptom or sign for Hospital Medicine was produced by the lesion and consequently could be used to infer the existence and exact nature of the disease. Surveillance Medicine takes these discrete elements of symptom, sign and disease and subsumes them under a more general category of 'factor' that points to, though does not necessarily produce, some future illness. Such inherent contingency is embraced by the novel and pivotal medical concept of *risk*. It is no longer the symptom or sign pointing tantalisingly at the hidden pathological truth of disease, but the risk factor opening up a space of future illness potential.

Symptoms and signs are only important for Surveillance Medicine to the extent that they can be re-read as risk factors. Equally, the illness in the form of the disease or lesion that had been the end-point of clinical inference under Hospital Medicine is also deciphered as a risk factor in as much as one illness becomes a risk factor for another. Symptom, sign, investigation and disease thereby become conflated into an infinite chain of risks. A headache may be a risk factor for high blood pressure (hypertension), but high blood pressure is simply a risk factor for another illness (stroke). And whereas symptoms, signs and diseases were located in the body, the risk factor encompasses any state or event from which a probability of illness can be calculated. This means that Surveillance Medicine turns increasingly to an extracorporal space – often represented by the notion of 'lifestyle' – to identify the precursors of future illness. Lack of exercise and a high fat diet therefore can be joined with angina, high blood cholesterol and diabetes as risk factors for heart disease. Symptoms, signs, illnesses, and health behaviours simply become indicators for yet other symptoms, signs, illnesses and health behaviours. Each illness of Hospital Medicine existed as the discrete endpoint in the chair of clinical discovery: in Surveillance Medicine each illness is simply a nodal point in a network of health status monitoring. The problem is less illness *per se* but the semi-pathological pre-illness at-risk state.

Under Hospital Medicine the symptom indicated the underlying lesion in a static relationship; true, the 'silent' lesion could exist without indicating its presence but eventually the symptomatic manifestations erupted into clinical consciousness. The risk factor, however, has no fixed nor necessary relationship with future illness, it simply opens up a space of possibility. Moreover, the risk factor exists in a mobile relationship with other risks, appearing and disappearing, aggregating and disaggregating, crossing spaces within and without the corporal body.

In terms of secondary spatialisation Hospital Medicine operated within the three-dimensional corporal volume of the sick patient. In contrast, the risk factor network of Surveillance Medicine is read across an extra-corporal and temporal space. In part, the new space of illness is the community. Community space incorporates the physical agglomeration of buildings and homes and their concomitant risks to health, though risks from the physical environment reflect more on nineteenth century concerns with sanitation and hygiene (Armstrong 1993). Twentieth century surveillance begins to focus more on the grid of interactions between people in the community. This multifaceted population space encompasses the physical gap between bodies that needs constant monitoring to guard against transmission of contagious diseases, such as tuberculosis, venereal disease and childhood infections. But the space between bodies is also, from the early twentieth century, a psycho-social space which is marked by the shift in the psychiatric/medical gaze from the binary problem of insanity/sanity to the generalised population problems of the neuroses (which affect everyone) (Armstrong 1979), and the crystallisation of individual attitudes, beliefs, cognitions and behaviours, limits of self-efficacy, ecological concerns, and aspects of lifestyle that have become such a pre-occupation of progressive health care tactics.

References

Armstrong, D. (1979) Madness and coping, *Sociology of Health and Illness*, 2, 293–316.

Armstrong, D. (1983) *Political Anatomy of the Body: Medical Knowledge in Britain in the Twentieth Century*. Cambridge: Cambridge University Press.

Armstrong, D. (1987) Silence and truth in death and dying, *Social Science of Medicine*, 24, 651–7.

Armstrong, D. (1993) Public health spaces and the fabrication of identity, *Sociology*, 27, 393–410.

Brown, M. A. (1929) *Teaching Health in Fargo*. New York: Commonwealth Fund.

Fitzpatrick, R., Hinton, J., Newman, S., Scambler, G. and Thompson, J. (1984) *The Experience of Illness*. London: Tavistock.

Foucault, M. (1973) *The Birth of the Clinic: An Archaeology of Medical Perception*. London: Tavistock.

HMSO (1975). *The School Health Service: 1908–74*. London: HMSO.

Kagawa-Singer, M. (1993) Redefining health: living with cancer, *Social Science and Medicine*, 37, 295–304.

Last, J. M. (1963) The clinical iceberg, *Lancet*, 2, 28–30.

Mechanic, D. and Volkart, E. H. (1960) Illness behaviour and medical diagnoses, *Journal of Health and Human Behaviour*, 1, 86–90.

Pearse, I. H. and Crocker, L. H. (1943) *The Peckham Experiment: A Study in the Living Structure of Society*. London: George Allen and Unwin.

Pickering, G. (1962) Logic and hypertension, *Lancet*, 2, 149.

Rose, N. (1985) *The Psychological Complex*. London: Routledge and Kegan Paul.

Rose, N. (1990) *Governing the Soul: The Shaping of the Private Self*. London: Routledge.

Smith, F. B. (1979) *The People's Health: 1830–1910*. London: Croom Helm.

20 The diagnostic test and the danger within*

Deborah Lupton

The current popularity of testing and screening procedures to diagnose disease in its early stages is a modernist response to the threat of disease and death, especially that which lurks invisibly in the body. The ill or diseased body often no longer announces its condition in luridly visible ways: pathology has become reduced to the invisible workings of cells, lymphocytes, bacteria and viruses. To detect this silent illness, a diagnostic test is put forward as the solution. Concordant with the ideology of rationality which permeates biomedical discourses and practices, it is believed important to have 'knowledge' of the presence of a hidden illness within rather than remain ignorant, for such knowledge is viewed as allowing medical science the opportunity to step in (Herzlich and Pierret, 1987: 94; Nelkin and Tancredi, 1989). The discourse of diagnostic testing and screening represents these procedures as 'scientific' and objective, value-free determinations of a reality uncontaminated by social processes: 'The test is seen as an isolated event in which objective *technical* data rationally persuades patients of their normality thus *determining* the benefit, reassurance' (Daly, 1989: 100, emphasis in the original).

However a diagnosis based on a medical test is not a purely objective, technical event, but relies upon the social context of both doctor and patient, and may or may not be beneficial for the patient. Human error is also a factor which is ignored: in some diagnostic tests, the margin for human error is rather large, beginning from when the doctor or other health professional takes the sample of tissue/urine/blood or an X-ray. Test results are then constructed by laboratory technicians, who must carry out the test and, more importantly, *interpret* the result using subjective criteria often based on a continuum, such as colour change, shape of cells, degree of 'abnormality' and so forth. The possibility of receiving a false positive or false negative result, therefore, is quite high for some diagnostic tests, but this caveat is rarely conveyed to those undergoing the procedure (Edwards and Hall, 1992: 267). When the potential for false results is revealed to members of the public, they

*This is an extract from Lupton, D. (1995) *The Imperative of Health: Public Health and the Regulated Body*, Sage, pp. 92–9.

often react with anger and cynicism, having been assured that the process of undergoing the test would protect them from harm. One example is the controversy initiated in the Australian news media in late 1992 concerning the efficacy of Pap smear tests (used to detect the early stages of cervical cancer). News media reports drew attention to the advertising of the New South Wales Cancer Council, which had distributed posters of smiling women saying, 'Cancer of the cervix. It can't happen to me. I have a regular Pap test', suggesting that regular participation in the testing programme would ensure that women would never fall victim to the disease. The media reported several case studies of women who had undertaken regular Pap tests which gave negative results, but yet were later diagnosed with cervical cancer, some of whom had subsequently died. These stories provoked such front-page headlines as 'Revealed: Pap smears give the all-clear to many with cancer' (*Sydney Morning Herald*, 19 September 1992).

The experience of undergoing a diagnostic screening test is primarily an emotive one. Health promotion campaigns, in their efforts to persuade as many members of the target group as possible to attend for testing, attempt psychological manipulation by appealing to people's emotions, fears, anxieties and guilt feelings. They often focus upon the central notion of risk around which dramatic imagery of doom, death and fear are constructed (as will be shown in Chapter 4, anti-smoking and AIDS education campaigns have often adopted this approach). Anxiety about the disease is deliberately engendered by the inducements used to persuade individuals to attend such programmes, where previously none may have existed. Symptomless people are forced to consider the possibility of harbouring a serious disease. For example, in the attempt to recruit women for breast cancer screening programmes, health promotion literature tends to make the misleading suggestion that 'no women needs to die of breast cancer if she reads and heeds the leaflets of the cancer societies and has her breasts examined regularly' (Skrabanek, 1985: 316). The poster used to promote Pap smears discussed earlier used a similar strategy. Such exhortations often imply that not to do so is to let both the woman herself (that is, her body), as well as society, down. It is the woman's responsibility to attend for screening, and to attend regularly, or otherwise be held responsible for allowing the unchecked spread of cancer in her body. Women are invited to participate in breast cancer screening programmes without being given adequate information about the uncertainties and risks involved, and without being informed that their participation is required for further testing of the hypothesis that mammography works (Skrabanek, 1989: 428). Skrabanek (1985: 316) points out after an extensive review of the literature that the medical evidence is overwhelming that most forms of breast cancer are incurable, and that early detection therefore only adds years of anxiety and fear (see also, Roberts, 1989; Skrabanek, 1989). Healthy women are exhorted to attend mammographic screening programmes or to conduct breast self examination, only to be faced with a diagnosis which changes their lives but does not necessarily ameliorate their state of health.

Such emotional manipulation has also been taken up by commercial services attempting to attract customers. In Australia, a print media advertisement for a medical insurance fund advertises its mammographic screening service by asserting that: 'For many women early detection can mean a complete cure. Early detection is your best protection from the consequences of breast cancer. It can save your life, often without the need for a mastectomy.' The bright assurances of the value of mammographic screening in such advertising does not reveal the medical uncertainties around the efficacy of mammographic screening and subsequent treatment of breast lesions referred to above. In the United States, medical services are marketed to healthy women (who would otherwise have no need for medical services) using a language and style that mimic that of the women's health movement by emphasizing the demystification of medical technology and the right of all women to have access to health care services and to be actively involved. Thus the discourse of prevention, although positioned by women's health groups as a way of reducing women's dependence upon medical services, is often cynically used as a marketing device to attract female clients to such services as mammography screening, stress management courses, bone density screening for osteoporosis and hormone replacement therapy, most of which involve participation in expensive medical services rather than the prevention of ill-health (Whatley and Worcester, 1989: 200).

While screening is often promoted as a means of providing reassurance for individuals, this is not necessarily the case. Screening for any disease invariably engenders psychological costs among those screened in terms of the generation of high anxiety levels (Marteau, 1990: 26). Participants are told that the procedure is 'low risk', but they are not told of the high risk of psychological distress (Fentiman, 1988: 1042). In the clinical context, a false negative is more serious than a false positive result, for an individual who has been reassured that they have no signs of disease may be lost to the health system at a critical point, while false positive results can be rectified through follow-up tests. However, for the individual involved, a false positive result has potentially damaging psychological costs (Nelkin and Tancredi, 1989: 46–7). For some participants, receiving an invitation to be screened is enough to induce anxiety. Some participants may be more anxious after screening than before, even if they have received a normal test result. For those whose test is uncertain and requires further investigation, distress is an understandable reaction, and anxieties 'may remain for months or even years after a false positive result' (Marteau, 1990: 26). These observations of stress and anxiety in symptomless patients who are encouraged to attend screening raise serious doubts concerning the desirability of such programmes.

Daly, for example, examined the use of an echocardiology (cardiac ultrasound) test given to patients to 'reassure' them that their hearts were normal. She notes that echocardiology does not resolve uncertainty, for it requires 'interpretation of a complex moving image according to sometimes uncertain professional criteria' (1989: 104). Clinical diagnosis can contradict the test result; it is up to the cardiologist to decide what credence should be placed on the test. The cardiologist's decision may be coloured, consciously or sub-consciously, by a number of factors, including his or her dependence upon insurance referrals and the training he or she has received in interpreting test results (1989: 109). Thus, while patients subscribe to the notion that technological investigation of symptoms provides an objective diagnosis, the medical discourse obscures the social forces shaping the test result. For example, when patients have cardiac symptoms, the result of the test is used as a placebo to reassure them that there is nothing wrong, obscuring the lack of skill in directly diagnosing or treating cardiac symptoms with no clear organic cause (1989: 114). Unfortunately, rather than being reassured, many patients are left with considerably more doubts about their hearts as a direct result of having the test done.

Prenatal screening tests have become extremely popular as a means of alleviating prospective parents' fears about the normality of the foetus, and as such have largely been accepted as accurate and harmless. The routinization and wide acceptance of prenatal screening methods such as amniocentesis and ultrasound, however, have not taken into full account the relative risks and benefits of the techniques. For example, there is an almost 1 per cent risk of spontaneous abortion following an amniocentesis test, compared with a 2 per cent chance that there will be a genetic abnormality (Rapp, 1988). Such techniques serve to individualize the reasons for chromosomal abnormalities, locating them on the individual or couple and ignoring the wider social reasons that may have caused genetic changes, such as exposure to environ-mental tetragens (Hubbard, 1984). There is also a risk of irradiation of the foetus using ultrasound, the effects of which have not yet been fully studied because of its popularity. There is no evidence that routine ultrasound screening is beneficial to the health of infants, while some studies have suggested that there may be possible harmful effects such as the restriction of growth after multiple ultrasounds (Rowland, 1992: 69–70; Saul, 1994). Furthermore, having the procedure is not necessarily reassuring for potential parents: there have been several occasions in which ultrasound screening has provided false positive results, so that women have been told that the foetus is dead, or has a malformation, when in fact there has been no such problem. The implications of such results for mental anguish in pregnant women and their partners are obvious (Saul, 1994: 14). Such screening procedures also serve to construct the mother–foetal relationship in certain ways, representing the foetus as separate from the mother, and placing pressure on the mother to undertake as many medical procedures as possible to ensure the health of the foetus.

One British study (French et al., 1982: 619) found that both attenders and non-attenders of a breast screening programme were anxious about the screening examination. A high percentage of non-attenders said that they felt that 'one should not go looking for trouble' and that they were afraid of cancer being found. A study of Scottish women (Maclean et al., 1984) found that the invitation to attend screening provoked worries on the part of the women they interviewed. Deep fear and concern about possible breast cancer were voiced by almost 40 per cent of their sample. The authors report that for their sample 'the entire philosophy of screening was foreign and they could see no point in searching for hidden, invisible ills within their bodies' (1984: 281). As these findings suggest, there is a difference between medical and lay definitions of the experience of a medical test such as a mammogram, ultrasound, amniocentesis or Pap smear. Medical and public health discourse argue that people benefit from having the peace of mind that comes from knowing that 'all is well', and adopt the rhetoric of evangelism to encourage people to 'come forward' to be 'saved' (Posner, 1991: 172), yet people attend for screening in the hope that there will be no sign of disease.

When there is an abnormal finding, the result is a psychological shock as the individual changes identity from a well person to a person harbouring disease. In two studies of British women undergoing screening for cervical cancer (Posner and Vessey, 1988; Quilliam, 1990), it was found that if there is occasion for further diagnostic procedures, waiting for and undergoing colposcopy (a surgical procedure to aid diagnosis of cervical cancer) can entail several months of agonized waiting for the woman and her family before she is told whether or not she really does have the disease. During this time, the women interviewed experienced a variety of emotions and thought processes including self-blame, sexual guilt, feeling dirty, creating links with past sexual traumas such as rape or abortion, fears of infertility, fear of death, dependency on health professionals and guilt about emotions. The fear of cancer, for many women, was debilitating: women expressed a feeling of defilement, alienation and loss of control of their own bodies, and were anxious waiting for their treatment. These feelings are created by the cultural meanings of cervical cancer, produced partly from health education messages, surrounding the sexually transmitted nature of the human papilloma virus which, it is currently believed, is associated with cervical cancer. Added to this medical definition of the cause of cervical cancer is the fact that the cancer occurs at the site of female reproduction and sexual activity, a bodily organ considered dangerous, unclean and mysterious. The interviewed women described cervical cancer in extremely negative terms. For example, one woman spoke of a 'vision of a dirty, horrible festering growth festering inside you', while another described the disease as 'a black fungus, creeping, mouldy' (Posner and Vessey, 1988: 56). The lack of clarity surrounding diagnosis of a pre-cancerous condition of the cervix is confusing and distressful for women. There are no certain explanations for the causes of a positive smear, so women cannot come to terms with why it happened to them. Furthermore, the alleged link with sexual activity may create doubt about their partner's fidelity, or incur hostility on the part of their partner.

These issues are also highly relevant to HIV antibody testing. The current irrational discrimination, fear and prejudice levelled against people with HIV/AIDS is a prime example of the way in which being 'at risk' becomes the equivalent of sinning. Research undertaken by McCombie (1986) illustrates the moral meanings around risk assessment and HIV antibody testing. She studied the counselling given by health workers to individuals deemed either 'high risk' or 'low risk' after an HIV test had been performed. McCombie noticed that 'high risk' individuals, whether HIV positive or negative, were treated differently from 'low risk' individuals: 'the high risk person is chastized, admonished and warned, while the low risk person is consoled and reassured' (1986: 455). She evaluated this behaviour in the context of taboo violation, pollution and punishment for sin. 'High risk' individuals were being punished for their deviant behaviour and were held responsible for their own behaviour if positive. By contrast, individuals deemed at low risk were looked upon more as innocent victims. The blood test itself was a ritual, acting as an anxiety-reducing measure for those who were concerned that the virus was getting out of control as well as implicitly acting as a tool for detecting social deviance.

Goldstein (1989: 89) views the process of having an HIV antibody test as an act 'of enormous courage', and asserts that in taking the test, people 'pass through a psychic rite that has less to do with fear of death than with the consequences of a positive result: guilt over the past, rage at the present, fear of the future. That fear must include not only the disease but disclosure – and the range of rejections that might ensue.' The experience of being identified as HIV positive can be personally destructive and almost inevitably emotionally harrowing (Grimshaw, 1987). Individuals who test positive will probably have to struggle with the imminent threat of death for the rest of their lives (notwithstanding the current controversy over the thesis that HIV is the cause of AIDS, discussed earlier in this chapter). Furthermore, there is a strong stigma associated with seropositivity and many members of the population are less sympathetic towards people living with HIV/AIDS than they are towards people with other conditions or illnesses. People living with HIV/AIDS are open to discrimination in the workforce, health care setting and other areas of life. For women who are pregnant or planning pregnancy there are associated anxieties, including the likelihood of transferring infection to the infant and the possibility of being abandoned by the father of the child should seropositivity be identified (Almond and Ulanowsky, 1990).

There has been very little research conducted into the reasons why people decide to participate in medical tests such as the HIV antibody test which throws light on the symbolic use of testing. In a study carried out by myself and colleagues (Lupton et al., 1995a, 1995b), people living in Sydney who had had at least one HIV antibody test were interviewed concerning their reasons for having a test and their experiences of the testing procedure. It was found that although the majority of the respondents had not engaged in the highest risk activities for contracting HIV, according to epidemiological orthodoxies current at the time (for example unprotected anal sex or sharing needles to inject drugs), many were using the test as a way of protecting their body boundaries from invasion and re-establishing subjectivity and feelings of self-containment after having sexual encounters. As one of the participants (a 26-year-old male) put it: 'I think if you're going to be sticking parts of your body into someone else or letting someone stick parts of their body into you, then you've got every right to make sure that the bits they stick in aren't going to leave something when they're gone.' For some interviewees, the test represented a disciplinary procedure, in which participants punished themselves for their lack of control over their bodies. The test was also used to punish others (one's unfaithful sexual partners) when the revelation of their infidelity came to light, or as a way of establishing purity, before launching into another relationship. People spoke of the need to 'clean the slate' at the end of a relationship and justified it in terms of their responsibility to protect themselves or their prospective partners from any diseases that may have been transmitted by the previous partner. They explained that having the test confirm their HIV status at the end of a relationship was the last phase in the closing process that accompanies many relationships and, subsequently, heralded a new beginning for them. For many participants, offering to take the test was a way of demonstrating their sense of responsibility and commitment to their partner. Others, particularly men, had the test only because they were under duress from their partner, or wanted to dispense with condom use, while some people seemed to see the HIV test as part of a general health care maintenance programme, in which one had a regular test along with screens such as Pap smears or cholesterol tests. The assumption was that a positive result, indicating the presence of a condition or disease, was very unlikely. For many of the participants, therefore, the HIV antibody test was symbolically acting as a preventive rather than a diagnostic measure.

As these findings suggest, the discourses and meanings surrounding the experience of taking a diagnostic test may be very different for participants compared with the 'official' interpretation of the process. Those individuals whose anxiety is aroused by having a test will not always be reassured by the result, and may find the experience degrading and frightening, placing them in a liminal state where they are neither 'ill' nor 'well'. Others may seek testing for reasons other than wanting to discern the presence of disease. Diagnostic tests may be used symbolically as almost magical rituals, conceptualized as protecting individuals from the disease or acting as a purifying rite. Alternatively, they may be used for such purposes as proving commitment to a relationship.

References

Almond, B. and Ulanowsky , C. (1990) HIV and pregnancy. *Hastings Center Report*, March/April, pp. 16–21.

Daly, J. (1989) Innocent murmurs: echocardiography and the diagnosis of cardiac normality. *Sociology of Health and Illness*, 11(2), 99–116.

Edwards, P.J. and Hall, D.M.B. (1992) Screening, ethics, and the law. *British Medical Journal*, 305, 267–8.

Fentiman, S. (1988) Pensive women, painful vigils: consequences of delay in assessment of mammographic abnormalities. *Lancet*, i, 1041–2.

French, K., Porter, A.M.D., Robinson, S.E., McCallum, F.M., Hoie, J.G.R. and Roberts, M.M. (1982) Attendance at a breast screening clinic: a problem of administration or attitudes. *British Medical Journal*, 285, 617–20.

Goldstein, R (1989) AIDS and the social contract. In Carter, E. and Watney, S. (eds), *Taking Liberties: AIDS and Cultural Politics*. London: Serpent's Tail, pp. 81–94.

Grimshaw, J. (1987) Being HIV antibody positive. *British Medical Journal*, 295, 256–7.

Herzlich, C. and Pierret, J. (1987) *Illness and Self in Society*. Baltimore, MD: Johns Hopkins University Press.

Hubbard, R. (1984) Personal courage is not enough: some hazards of childbearing in the 1980s. In Arditti, R., Klein, R.D. and Minden, S. (eds), *Test-tube Women: What Future for Motherhood?* London: Pandora, pp. 331–55.

Lupton, D., McCarthy, S. and Chapman, S. (1995a) 'Panic bodies': discourses on risk and HIV antibody testing. *Sociology of Health and Illness*, 17(1), 89–108.

Lupton, D., McCarthy, S. and Chapman, S. (1995b) 'Doing the right thing': the symbolic meanings and experiences of having an HIV antibody test. *Social Science and Medicine*, 41(2), 173–80.

McCombie, S. (1986) The cultural impact of the 'AIDS' test: the American experience. *Social Science and Medicine*, 23(5), 455–9.

Maclean, U., Sinfield, D., Klein, S. and Harnden, B. (1984) Women who decline breast screening. *Journal of Epidemiology and Community Health*, 38, 278–83.

Marteau, T.M. (1990) Reducing the psychological costs. *British Medical Journal*, 310, 26–8.

Nelkin, D. and Tancredi, L. (1989) *Dangerous Diagnostics: the Social Power of Biological Information*. New York: Basic Books.

Posner, T. (1991) What's in a smear? Cervical screening, medical signs and metaphors. *Science as Culture*, 2(2), 167–87.

Posner, T. and Vessey, M. (1988) *Prevention of Cervical Cancer: the Patient's View*. London: King Edward's Hospital Fund for London.

Quilliam, S. (1990) Positive smear: the emotional issues and what can be done. *Health Education Journal*, 49(1), 19–20.

Rapp, R. (1988) Chromosomes and communication: the discourse of genetic counselling. *Medical Anthropology Quarterly*, 2(2), 143–57.

Roberts, M.M. (1989) Breast screening: time for a rethink? *British Medical Journal*, 299, 1153–4.

Rowland, R. (1992) *Living Laboratories: Woman and Reproductive Technologies*. Sydney: Pan Macmillan.

Saul, H. (1994) Screening without meaning? *New Scientist*, 19 March, 14–15.

Skrabanek, P. (1985) False premises and false promises of breast cancer screening. *Lancet*, ii, 316–20.

Skrabanek, P. (1989) Mass mammography: time for a reappraisal. *International Journal of Technology Assessment in Health Care*, 5, 423–30.

Whatley, M.H. and Worcester, N. (1989) The role of technology in the co-optation of the women's health movement: the cases of osteoporosis and breast cancer screening. In Ratcliff, K.S., Ferree, M.M., Mellow, G.O., Wright, B.D., Price, G.D., Yanoshik, K. and Freston, M.S. (eds), *Healing Technology: Feminist Perspectives*. Ann Arbor, MI: University of Michigan Press, pp. 199–220.

21 The modern rise of population*

Thomas McKeown

Since the conclusions concerning the modern rise of population have been developed over several chapters, it will be desirable to bring them together in a general interpretation. I will begin by summarizing some of the main points made in the preceding pages.

When the rise of population from the eighteenth century to the present day is considered as a whole – and there are compelling reasons for this approach – it is seen to be a unique event which cannot be explained in the same terms as earlier population increases. Something happened which led to a greater and more prolonged expansion of population than any which preceded it.

The expansion was not due to an increase in the birth rate brought about by withdrawal of restraints on fertility. There is no evidence of this in developing countries today, or in developed countries since births and deaths were recorded reliably by national registration; indeed for most of the time birth rates have been falling. [. . .] The increase of population is therefore attributable to a decline of mortality.

The decline of mortality was due essentially to a reduction of deaths from infectious diseases. National statistics show this to be the reason for the decline in England from registration (in 1838) until 1900, and it remains the pre-dominant influence to the present day. It seems reasonable to conclude that the fall of mortality in the eighteenth and early nineteenth centuries was also associated with the infectious diseases, although it is probable that there was a substantial decrease of deaths from two non-infective causes, infanticide and starvation. [. . .]

The fall of mortality was not influenced substantially by immunization or therapy before 1935 when sulphonamides became available. This conclusion is based both on knowledge of the role of medical measures in the present day, and consideration of the reasons for the decline of the major diseases which were associated with the reduction of mortality. The decrease of deaths from infections in which specific medical measures were effective earlier than 1935

*This is an abridged extract from McKeown, T. (1976) *The Modern Rise of Population*, Edward Arnold, pp. 152–4, 158–62.

– smallpox, syphilis, tetanus, diphtheria, diarrhoeal diseases and some surgical conditions – made only a small contribution to the total decline of the death rate after 1838.

Exclusion of a fortuitous change in the character of infectious diseases and of immunization and therapy leaves one other explanation for the reduction of mortality, namely, improvements in the environment. The questions remain whether there are positive as well as negative grounds for this conclusion, and whether it is possible to specify the nature of the environmental influences.

From the second half of the nineteenth century a substantial reduction of mortality from intestinal infections followed the introduction of hygienic measures – purification of water, efficient sewage disposal and improved food hygiene, particularly in respect of milk. It is unlikely that such influences were effective before that time, since initially industrialization led to crowding and deterioration of hygienic conditions. However, the decline of infectious diseases which occurred progressively from the eighteenth century must have resulted in reduced contact with some infections as a secondary consequence of the diminished prevalence of the diseases.

The most acceptable explanation of the large reduction of mortality and growth of population which preceded advances in hygiene is an improvement in nutrition due to greater food supplies. The grounds for this conclusion are twofold. (a) There was undoubtedly a great increase in food production during the eighteenth and nineteenth centuries, in England and Wales enough to support a population which trebled between 1700 and 1850 without significant food imports. (b) In the circumstances which existed prior to the agricultural and industrial revolutions, an improvement in food supplies was a necessary condition for a substantial and prolonged decline of mortality and expansion of population. The last point is in accord with present-day knowledge of the relation between malnutrition and infectious diseases.

The decline of mortality from non-infective causes of death (infanticide and starvation in the eighteenth and nineteenth centuries and a large number of conditions in the twentieth) was due partly to medical measures, but also to contraception and improvement in nutrition. Indeed, since the reduction of deaths from infanticide probably made the largest contribution to the decline, the change in reproductive behaviour which resulted in avoidance of unwanted pregnancies was probably the most important influence on the decrease of deaths from non-infective conditions. [. . .]

In the light of these conclusions it is not difficult to interpret the reasons for the predominance of infectious diseases during the past 10,000 years.

The increase in food supplies which resulted from the first agricultural revolution led to the growth of populations to the size and density needed for the propagation and transmission of micro-organisms. However, as the population continued to expand, food resources became again marginal, so that the relation between man and micro-organisms evolved over a period when man was, in general, poorly nourished. The relationship was unstable and finely balanced according to the physiological state of host and parasite;

improvement in nutrition would tip the balance in favour of the former and deterioration in favour of the latter. In these circumstances an increase in food supplies became a necessary condition for a substantial reduction of mortality from infectious diseases, and limitation of numbers would have to follow if the reduction was to be made permanent.

These were the critical advances made in the western world in the eighteenth and nineteenth centuries. From about the end of the seventeenth century there was an enormous increase in food production, in Britain sufficient to feed a population which trebled between 1700 and 1850 with little supplement from imported foods. [. . .]

Yet the improvement in health which resulted from the advances in agriculture would in time have been reversed, as that which presumably followed the first agricultural revolution was reversed, by increasing numbers, if the growth of population had not been restricted. But in France from the beginning of the nineteenth century, and in other countries somewhat later, the birth rate began to decline. In the same period food supplies continued to increase, and together the two influences maintained the favourable balance between food and numbers. Hence we owe the reduction of mortality and growth of population basically to improved nutrition which resulted from the increase in food and to the change in reproductive behaviour which ensured that the advance was not reversed.

The other major influence on the trend of the infections was reduction of exposure. As a primary influence, this was delayed until the second half of the nineteenth century, when men began to improve the quality of the environment. The initial advances were the purification of water, efficient disposal of sewage, and food hygiene, which together led to a rapid decline of intestinal diseases spread by water and food. Such measures had no effect on exposure to airborne infections, the diseases mainly associated with the reduction of mortality during the nineteenth century. However, in a period when infectious diseases are declining, for whatever reason, less frequent exposure follows as a secondary consequence of their reduced prevalence in the community. It is therefore probable that in the eighteenth and nineteenth centuries exposure to some infections decreased, as clearly it has in the case of tuberculosis in the twentieth century.

For the population as a whole this improvement secondary to lower prevalence must have been offset largely by deteriorating environmental conditions associated with industrialization; the crowding at home and at work in the industrial towns created ideal conditions for the spread of air-borne diseases, and no doubt contributed substantially to the predominance of tuberculosis as a cause of death in the nineteenth century. But for the well-to-do, the advantages of reduced exposure as a secondary consequence of the lower prevalence of infectious diseases were not offset by deteriorating working and living conditions. This may explain, at least in part, the observation that life expectation of the aristocracy increased in the eighteenth and nineteenth centuries, although they would be expected to offer little scope for the main influence on the general population, namely, an improvement in nutrition.

Finally, I must consider the part played by medical measures of immunization and therapy, long thought to be the main reason for population growth in the eighteenth century, and still considered significant by those attracted by the idea that inoculation led to a reduction of deaths from smallpox. In relation to the increase of population in the past three centuries the issue arises particularly in respect of the infections for, with the important exceptions of infanticide and starvation, until the twentieth century the decline of mortality was associated almost wholly with infectious diseases.

These are three lines of evidence which have led to the conclusion that medical measures had relatively little effect on the trend of mortality from the infections. First, there is increasing recognition that health is determined essentially by behavioural and environmental influences, and that the scope for effective medical intervention is limited. This is true not only of infections, but also of diseases such as cancer, chronic bronchitis and certain forms of heart disease, formerly thought to be intractable and now shown to be largely preventable by modification of behaviour and of the environment.

The second kind of evidence is derived from experience in developing countries, where it has been found that nutritional state is critical in determining the frequency and outcome of the infections. This is true even of diseases such as measles and whooping cough for which effective immunization is available, and indeed it is questionable whether infectious diseases can be controlled by immunization in a malnourished population.

The third line of enquiry has an even more direct bearing on assessment of the influence of immunization and therapy on the trend of mortality from infectious diseases in the period when they can be identified in national statistics, in Britain from the fourth decade of the nineteenth century. Examination of the diseases mainly associated with the fall of mortality shows that their death rates declined long before the introduction of effective immunization or treatment, and that by the time these measures became available the rates had fallen to a relatively low level. The diseases in which effective vaccination or therapy were available in the nineteenth or early twentieth centuries made only a small contribution to the reduction of mortality; it was not until 1935, with the introduction of sulphonamides and later, antibiotics, that medical measures became available which were sufficiently powerful to have an effect on national death rates. And even since 1935 they have not been the only or, probably, the main influences. [. . .]

The great increase in food production from the end of the seventeenth century resulted in improvement in nutrition, and tipped the balance in favour of the hosts and against micro-organisms which cause disease. At this time however, and unlike experience 10,000 years earlier, numbers did not rise to the point at which food supplies again became marginal; food production continued to increase by the application of technology to agriculture; and even more important, population growth was limited by falling birth rates.

The greatly expanded populations of the industrial towns created ideal conditions for the spread of infectious diseases. The fact that mortality from the diseases declined in spite of these conditions indicates the critical influence of nutrition; a population which was fed better, if not adequately, was able to face the risks of increased exposure. Moreover, exposure to infection was limited in two ways: one indirect, as a result of the lower prevalence of the diseases; the other direct, following improvement in hygiene of water and food from the second half of the nineteenth century. The protection of milk was particularly important, for milk provides an excellent medium for the growth of micro-organisms and was largely responsible for the high level of infant mortality which continued until 1900.

There need be no disappointment with the conclusion that medical measures of immunization and treatment were relatively ineffective; they were also unnecessary. In the classical tradition there were two ideas concerning man's health: one, associated with the goddess Hygieia, that it could be achieved by a rational way of life; the other, personified by the god Asclepius, that it depended largely on the role of the physician as healer of the sick. Both concepts are to be found in Hippocratic writings, and they have survived in medical thought and practice down to the present day. However, since the seventeenth century at least, the Asclepian approach has been predominant. Philosophically, it derived support from Descartes' concept of the living organism as a machine which might be taken apart and reassembled if its structure and function were understood; practically, it seemed to find confirmation in the work of Kepler and Harvey and in the success of the physical sciences in manipulating inanimate matter. It is only in the past few decades that it has become evident that this interpretation is quite inaccurate, that the health of man is determined essentially by his behaviour, his food and the nature of the world around him, and is only marginally influenced by personal medical care. Intuitively we believe that *we are ill and are made well*; it is nearer the truth to say that *we are well and are made ill.*

22 From tribalism to corporatism

The managerial challenge to medical dominance*

David J. Hunter

It has already been suggested that the medical profession has a rather odd relationship with the NHS, in particular the lack of a sense of belonging to a broader organisational entity. This leads one to wonder whether, despite many individual exceptions, the profession's attachment to the NHS is largely one of convenience or necessity rather than genuine commitment. The sense of attachment or belonging to an organisation could be seen as of negligible importance for the profession as a whole.

Arising from this perception of the relationship of doctors to the NHS are a number of barriers that preserve a tribalistic mode of operating rather than promote a corporate or collaborative one. The separatist nature of clinical work is reinforced by a particular interpretation of the doctor–patient relationship. The notion of 'possessive individualism' results in doctors functioning independently not only of the rest of the organisation but also of each other. This occurs despite the alleged collegiate nature of their organisation, which remains true in an overall collective sense but is less apparent at the level of inter-specialty relations. The education of doctors and the position of the Royal Colleges reinforce barriers and elitism. Postgraduate medical education continues to foster the isolation of specialties from each other. The hierarchical nature of medicine in respect of its internal stratification between consultants and junior doctors and between specialties makes it more likely that vertical relationships figure over and above horizontal ones (Hunter *et al.* 1988). There is less commitment to an integrated approach across specialties, professions and agencies as a consequence. The concept of 'interface management' between specialties is not highly valued and doctors receive little training in negotiating and team building skills (Hunter 1990). Indeed, medical education with its compartmentalised approach to modern medicine almost encourages fragmentation. It certainly institutionalises it.

There are countervailing forces at play which provide a destabilising influence as far as tribalism is concerned. A greater degree of corporatism may be the outcome. First, there is the effect of the NHS reforms. The purchaser–

*This is an extract from a chapter first published in Gabe, J., Kelleher, D. and Williams, G. (eds) (1994) *Challenging Medicine*, Routledge, pp. 1–22.

provider split has required providers to market their services and become more customer-oriented. Hospitals with trust status cannot assume that business will automatically fall to them if the price and quality of care are unsatisfactory. As a result, they are having to evolve a corporate culture which can only succeed if doctors are a central part of it. As the survival of the hospital may be at stake there are strong externally derived pressures on doctors and managers to sink any differences which may exist between them and to act together to ensure the long-term viability of the services being provided.

Managers are increasingly reliant on clinical directors to run services and deliver the clinicians' commitment to tighter management of their work. Clinical directorates, through which doctors play a significant role in management, are maturing, although what their long-term prognosis is in terms of involving doctors in management is not known. The evidence from studies of clinical directorates suggests that some are working more effectively than others. A great deal appears to depend on the skills, interests and personalities of the particular individuals appointed as directors. Possibly the most sensitive issue has been that clinical directors are supposed to have a management role in relation to their consultant colleagues which has not, in practice, proved easy to realise (Fitzgerald 1991). There appears on the surface to be considerable support both for the appointment of doctors as clinical directors and the development of management budgets. Hitherto, this support has come principally from non-medical general managers, i.e. the agents of government, rather than doctors themselves, with the exception of a few converts. There must be limits on how supportive non-medical general managers will continue to be when they begin to realise that by encouraging doctors to enter management they may be putting their own careers at risk or those of their successors.

As long as there exists suspicion and lack of trust between clinicians and managers it seems inconceivable that clinical directorates can function effectively. Scrivens (1988a, 1988b) found in a survey of doctors limited interest among them in management and in taking responsibility for budgets. She claims that a major effort is needed to persuade doctors of the importance of medical involvement in management. The assumption made is that it is 'a good thing' for doctors to be involved in management, as, indeed, Griffiths (1983) argued when he referred to them as the 'natural managers' in the NHS, but there is a need for clarity about both the level at which doctors are introduced to management and the purpose of their involvement.

The nub of the problem arising from the management–medicine interface is the different values upheld by those practising management and those practising medicine respectively. As Moore (1990) has put it, managerial values 'emphasise collaborative action, teamwork and collective achievement' (Moore 1990: 18). In contrast, medicine's values stress the individual, the assumption being that the doctor will work on behalf of the best interests of the individual patient. The medical profession's ideology is one of 'maximising rather than optimising . . . individually rather than collectively orientated, and behaving independently in action rather than interdependently' (ibid.).

The upshot of these developments and observations is the need for a repertoire of new skills which are principally concerned with the 'softer' side of management. These skills include an ability to listen, tolerance, keeping an open mind, a sense of humility, sharing responsibility and a preparedness to relinquish absolute professional autonomy. Perhaps more fundamentally is a need for management to establish itself as a distinct entity rather than as something which professions and politicians can in turn seek to dominate and manipulate for their own respective ends (Mark and Scott 1992). Management in the NHS is vulnerable and, somewhat paradoxically given the attention lavished upon it, susceptible to a takeover by doctors or politicians or both. The threat from the former could have particularly far-reaching consequences in terms of the future direction taken by the NHS and health policy. It is significant in this regard that whenever doctors are asked to comment on why they should participate in management, the reply is invariably along the lines of the following:

> Doctors must play a bigger part in managing the health service *to protect their clinical freedom*.
>
> (Smith *et al.* 1989: 311, emphasis added)

From a survey conducted by Parkhouse *et al.* (1988) on the views of doctors, similar responses were recorded. For example:

> Doctors *must* run the NHS.
>
> (Parkhouse *et al.* 1988: 25)

> Non-medical managers simply will not understand what health care is necessary.
>
> (ibid.)

In short, doctors should get involved in management not to hasten or collude in the erosion of their freedom and the privileges it brings to dictate what kind of medicine is practised but to ensure that the erosion is resisted.

Medicine and management: a possible scenario

As the above sections have suggested, all the indications are that the involvement of doctors in management will continue to grow in keeping with the mounting pressures on governments to contain costs, to hold doctors more accountable for what they do, to investigate the causes of clinical variation and to propose solutions to them, to address issues of efficacy in respect of medical interventions to ensure that only cost-effective ones and those of proven value get adopted, and to give closer attention to the whole issue of health outcomes and the impact of health care and medicine on these.

What remains less clear is how doctors will choose to make an impact, at what level in the health care system, and with what consequences for the future shape of health services. As was noted at the outset of this chapter, the managerial challenge to medicine may be absorbed or deflected by the profession in ways which could leave it virtually intact or even strengthened. It therefore becomes necessary to examine not so much what doctors *feel* about the various influences on them but rather to assess the impact of these on practitioners' behaviour.

Evidence from the United States demonstrates that interference strategies that result in managers dominating agendas at the expense of doctors are doomed to failure (Shortell *et al.* 1990). Such strategies have had to be adapted and managerial behaviour modified to ensure that clinicians subscribed to them and that confrontation between managers and doctors was avoided. Studies such as that by Shortell and his colleagues underline the importance of developing effective interfaces and collaborative working relationships between managers and clinicians.

Moreover, there is always a risk of the 'special relationship' which doctors enjoy with the general public being invoked, thereby enabling them to sidestep or simply ignore policy/management developments of which they may disapprove. There is little evidence to substantiate the view that the social place of medicine or its intellectual dominance have been substantially or irrevocably eroded.

That medical power is reinforced by cultural factors is of great significance and sets medicine apart from other activities. The medical profession, despite its having been slightly dented by some questioning of its practices and treatments, by the increase in medical negligence claims and by the growth of alternative medicine, continues to enjoy high social status and respect – much higher, according to social surveys, than either politicians or managers.

In a survey conducted recently to find out whether members of the public would prefer doctors, managers or politicians to determine priorities in health, the majority put their faith first in hospital consultants (61 per cent), then in GPs (49 per cent) and finally in managers (22 per cent) (Heginbotham 1993).

Nor is it only members of the general public who are culturally predisposed to accept the authority of doctors. Most groups of health service workers are similarly deferential though this may be lessening, as in the case of managers imbued with the 'Local Voices' (NHSME 1992) philosophy of involving the public in decisions about which treatments should take higher priority.

Although management and managers in health care systems may be in the ascendency, it remains possible nevertheless for the balance of power still to operate in favour of doctors, regardless of whether they remain outside the management system or become managers themselves. In this respect, Lukes's (1974) analysis of power, particularly his three-dimensional model, is persuasive. The third face of power allows for consideration of the many ways in which *potential issues* are kept out of politics. The use of power in this sense can occur in the absence of actual, observable conflict.

The standard objection to Lukes's position is that since by definition the third dimension of power involves B's values and preferences being shaped by A, there remains no observable conflict of values and therefore no observable exercise of power. It becomes difficult in such circumstances to demonstrate the third dimension empirically. Lukes defends his position by arguing that it is valid for an observer to make a judgement about the 'real' ('objective') interests of actors: to reach, for instance, a conclusion that B has been manipulated into adopting preferences which are actually against B's interests. Whilst this argument is valid, it requires careful usage. A classic indicator of the presence of third-face medical power is the phrase used by non-doctors: 'Doctor knows best' (Harrison *et al.* 1992).

Lukes's conceptualisation of power is helpful in illuminating and explaining the seeming paradox of the medical profession allegedly under attack and having its freedoms curbed on the one hand while, on the other, societal views about doctors, and their status, and about the nature of medicine and health care generally reinforce the prevailing orthodoxy and serve to blunt attempts to challenge it. Empirical evidence exists to support such a view as outlined below.

Cost containment measures over the years have been modest in their aspirations. They have not sought to challenge in any fundamental way whether the medical model or medical industrial complex, which constitutes the modern health care delivery infrastructure, is worthy of the enormous investment it receives. Even the recent emphasis on, and rather modest investment in, effectiveness research largely reflects the traditional standard of scientific medicine to demonstrate the clinical value of its modalities. Nowhere in the changes affecting medicine can one find a serious challenge to the hegemony of the medical perspective (Mechanic 1991).

According to Mechanic, the evidence is slim that doctors are losing their clinical autonomy. He does not deny that such an outcome remains a possibility but so far there has been no fundamental challenge to the medical model and whether it 'is worthy of the enormous social investment it receives' (Mechanic 1991: 495). Mechanic is not alone in reaching a view that runs counter to much of the prevailing policy analysis centred on the ascendency of managerialism. As Evans (1990) notes, doctors are granted extraordinary privileges and undertake special obligations in order that they can perform in ways which best meet patient needs. He queries the commitment on the part of policy makers and managers to utilise the evidence that is currently available in respect of clinical variations in practice.

The collusive relationship with the public, referred to above, has allowed medicine's conception of health and disease to remain dominant. The NHS remains patient-, not population-, centred and it is by no means self-evident that the health strategy as set out in the *Health of the Nation* will shift this focus, although it challenges the dominant biomedical model and existing distribution of resources, and is beginning to shape the language of policy priorities (DH 1991). The Government's health strategy marks the first time in Britain that an explicit attempt has been made to set targets in selected areas by which to achieve demonstrable and measurable improvements in health. But the extent of the political commitment to such a challenge to the prevailing biomedical orthodoxy remains far from clear. Suggestions that medicine is under siege by numerous hostile forces arrayed against it in the shape of assertive managers and policy makers are almost certainly premature. The odd skirmish may afford a victory or two for the invading forces but the real issue is one of *sustainability* and the successful engineering of a new balance of power in medicine that gives managers a dominant role.

The instrument of management is double-edged and could be used to further the assault on medical power or to blunt it. It is unclear whether involving doctors in management and encouraging them to become managers represents a serious attempt to address these issues and seek movement in areas where it has been singularly lacking, or whether it is seen by doctors as a way of staving off any real threat to their privileged position. Involving doctors more centrally and pivotally in the management function could institutionalise and entrench the very forces that are likely to prevent any attempt to move from a medical model of disease to a broader, societal conception of health and illness.

The reason why many doctors get involved in management in the first place is instructive. As was pointed out earlier, research shows that it is not in order to hasten, or collude in, the erosion of their freedom but rather to ensure that the erosion is resisted or halted (Hunter 1992). Doctors as managers, then, becomes a perfectly legitimate stratagem for ensuring that no fundamental challenge is mounted to their prevailing view of the world. If colonising the strange, and somewhat alien, world of management becomes the means for securing this then so be it.

Paradoxically, having charged down the management route intent upon deploying management innovations to control or reconfigure clinical practice, the Government may have unwittingly laid the foundations for a resurgence of professional power. Far from the managerial revolution in health care success-fully challenging the notion of 'provider capture', it will have unwittingly served to entrench it (Hunter 1992). If such a development occurs on a significant scale then the future status of lay, or non-medical, managers surely becomes an issue. As Mark and Scott (1992) argue, 'medical managerialism has profound implications for both present managers without clinical qualifications and future lay recruits to management in the NHS' (Mark and Scott 1992: 210).

Whatever the outcome of manoeuvrings between doctors and managers the parameters of the management agenda seem likely to remain medically defined. If a doctor is challenged to behave like his or her more efficient colleagues, the criteria of judgement are best *medical* practice and not *manage-ment* practice. In short, the new management thinking will be adopted by doctors and may lead to a re-establishing of professional power in health services which some observers, perhaps mistakenly and almost certainly prematurely, believe has been somewhat battered and bruised by the recent introduction of various management techniques designed to confront doctors and to weaken their clinical autonomy (Flynn 1992).

Doctors' trump card in this on-going struggle with policy makers is their hold over life and death. Unless managers and governments wish to become directly responsible for life and death decisions, doctors will continue to retain the upper hand in any contest with the advocates of efficiency and effectiveness. After all, they alone command public confidence in their judgement in such matters. Unless doctors lose the respect and loyalty of the public they will continue to possess considerable power to contain countervailing forces. Should public criticism of and disillusionment with medicine grow significantly, then governments and managers are likely to gain in confidence and challenge the power base of doctors. But in no health care system, including the British NHS, has this stage in the management–medicine relationship been reached. It remains unclear whether the British NHS, following what many regard as the most far-reaching reforms in its history, will provide the breakthrough. It is certainly seen as a test case to be carefully observed and systematically evaluated.

Conclusion

This chapter has sought to demonstrate that the proletarianisation of the medical profession as a result of the most recent management reform of the British NHS is far from complete and that doctors retain considerable influence over the allocation of resources at an operational level and over the continuing dominance of the health policy agenda. It is not denied that the position of doctors has changed and that they now have to justify and account for their actions in ways unthinkable a decade or so ago, or that the biomedical model is not under challenge as a result of a revival of the public health movement. But these forces have yet to play themselves out and it is by no means certain that doctors will have to surrender their position even if required to be more explicit about it or to share it with others in the health policy arena, or both. They could seek to maintain it.

While on the face of it developments in management and health policy can be seen to pose a major threat to medical dominance as it has traditionally been configured, the preceding analysis has sought to challenge this view by arguing that (a) the medical profession continues to enjoy high social standing, and (b) doctors may be resorting to countervailing sources of power to shape the new managerial developments to their agenda and definition of medical care. There are signs that this is already happening. For example, medical audit remains under the control of doctors despite its potential for giving managers a weapon to control ineffective doctors. It has been argued that the medical profession is more tribalistic than collegiate. An exception occurs when the profession is under threat or perceives itself to be so. Then a united front is put up as doctors combine against the common foe.

Another critical development which poses a threat to doctors lies in the R&D strategy and the new industry rapidly being built up in health services research, including outcomes research. But, for all the claims being confidently articulated in support of these developments, they could result in having a minimal impact overall on current practice if purchasing authorities in the new NHS remain weak and undeveloped or reluctant to challenge current orthodoxy and if the agenda continues to be driven by providers (Hunter and Harrison 1993). Similarly, the R&D initiative should in theory provide ammunition, in the form of empirical evidence concerning medical treatments and their effectiveness, for managers to challenge doctors. Whether it will actually function in this way depends on whether managers attach sufficient importance to R&D and whether doctors are prepared to change their practices in accordance with the research evidence. If the R&D strategy becomes captured by a biomedical perspective, as some predict, then it will most likely fail to effect real or lasting change in the NHS (Hunter 1993).

These two examples lead this writer to be wary of claims that the proletarianisation of medicine in the British NHS is all but complete and that medical power has been successfully harnessed by the advance of managerialism. The policy landscape in health care in Britain continues to shift and remains turbulent. It is by no means certain that the tenets of the 'new public management' will continue to hold sway. Mechanic and Evans's analyses of medical dominance are more persuasive at a time of uncertainty in which the confusion over managerial and medical roles is far from being resolved. More time needs to have elapsed before we can assert with any confidence, on the basis of reliable evidence, that medical dominance has been replaced with a particular managerial ethos. This may be a perfectly respectable and reasonable position to take but it also risks ignoring the considerable political skills of doctors who are adept at redirecting or neutralising attempts by governments and managers to control them. These skills may serve them well once again as they seek to resist the corporate embrace even if part of the strategy of resistance involves adopting the trappings of corporatism.

References

Department of Health (DH) (1991) *The Health of the Nation*, London: HMSO.

Evans, R.G. (1990) 'The day in the night-time: medical practice variations and health policy', in Mooney, G. and Andersen, T.S. (eds) *The Challenge of Medical Practice Variations*, Basingstoke: Macmillan.

Fitzgerald, L. (1991) 'Made to measure', *Health Service Journal*, 31 October: 24–5.

Flynn, R. (1992) *Structures of Control in Health Management*, London: Routledge.

Griffiths, R. (1983) *NHS Management Inquiry*, Report, London: DHSS.

Harrison, S., Hunter, D.J., Marnoch, G. and Pollitt, C. (1992) *Just Managing: Power and Culture in the National Health Service*, Basingstoke: Macmillan.

Heginbotham, C. (1993) *Healthcare Priority Setting: A Survey of Doctors, Managers and the General Public*, London: King's Fund College.

Hunter, D.J. (1990) 'Managing the cracks: management development for health care interfaces', *International Journal of Health Planning and Management*, 5(1): 7–14.

—— (1992) 'Doctors as managers: poachers turned gamekeepers?', *Social Science and Medicine*, 35(4): 557–66.

—— (1993) 'Let's hear it for R&D', *Health Service Journal*, 15 April: 17.

Hunter, D.J. and Harrison, S. (1993) *Effective Purchasing for Health Care: Proposals for First 5 Years*, Leeds: Nuffield Institute for Health.

Hunter, D.J., McKeganey, N.P. and MacPherson, I.A. (1988) *Care of the Elderly: Policy and Practice*, Aberdeen: Aberdeen University Press.

Lukes, S. (1974) *Power: A Radical View*, London: Macmillan.

Mark, A. and Scott, H. (1992) 'Management in the NHS', in Willcocks, L. and Harrow, J. (eds) *Rediscovering Public Services Management*, London: McGraw Hill.

Mechanic, D. (1991) 'Sources of countervailing power in medicine', *Journal of Health Politics, Policy and Law*, 16(3): 485–506.

Moore, G.T. (1990) 'Doctors as managers: frustrating tensions', in Costain, D. (ed.) *The Future of Acute Services: Doctors as Managers*, London: King's Fund Centre.

NHS Management Executive (1992) *Local Voices*, London: NHSME.

Parkhouse, J., Ellin, D.J. and Parkhouse, H.F. (1988) 'The views of doctors on management and administration', *Community Medicine*, 10: 19–32.

Scrivens, E. (1988a) 'Doctors and managers: never the twain shall meet?' *British Medical Journal*, 296: 1,754–6.

—— (1988b) 'The management of clinicians in the NHS', *Social Policy and Administration*, 22: 22–34.

Shortell, S., Morrison, E. and Friedman, B. (1990) *Strategic Choices for America's Hospitals*, New York: Jossey Bass.

Smith, R., Grabbam, A. and Chantler, C. (1989) 'Doctors becoming managers', *British Medical Journal*, 298: 311.

23 Disability and the myth of the independent researcher*

Colin Barnes

At a recent seminar on the relationship between medical sociology and disability theory I was struck by the response from some non-disabled and disabled academics to a call from a disabled delegate from an organisation of disabled people for guidelines on how to deal with requests from researchers for information and collaboration on disability-related research. Although the enquirer was clearly concerned about the ease with which researchers can easily misrepresent disability, those who responded used the request as an opportunity to put forward their own positions as independent researchers. They were concerned that in disability research, as in research generally, researchers must be free of all external considerations and controls in order to produce valid and unbiased results.

Now, given the history of disability research and the way that some disabled people have argued that it has played a role in the oppression of disabled people (see, for example, Hunt, 1981; Oliver, 1990, 1992; Morris, 1992; Abberley, 1992; Rioux and Bach, 1994), it seems quite understandable to me that disabled people and their organisations should be wary of researchers. What is more difficult to understand, however, is the way in which some academics continue to argue for the idea of the 'independent researcher' without qualification. In my view this is a strategy which is, at best, naïve and, at worst, misleading.

Setting aside the apparently never ending and seemingly irreconcilable debates about value freedom, 'objectivity' and appropriate methodologies within social science (see Pawson, 1989; Sayer, 1992), in Britain the myth of the independent researcher has its roots in the university system. Historically, British universities have fulfilled at least two main functions. Besides providing a particular form of advanced education for a certain section of the population, they have provided the necessary facilities for a select group of individuals to conduct research on a whole range of issues unfettered by the mundane demands of everyday life. Although this frequently abused privilege

*This article was first published in *Disability and Society*, vol. 11, no. 1, pp. 107–10, 1996, and subsequently in Barton, L., and Oliver, M. (eds) (1997) *Disability Studies: Past, Present and Future*, The Disability Press, pp. 239–43.

was almost exclusively reserved for the middle and upper classes, most universities, in accordance with their charitable status [*sic*] provided some form of support through sponsorship and bursaries for those considered worthy, but without.

Today, this tradition finds expression in postgraduate training programmes and fellowships sponsored by either Government funded research councils, such as the Economic and Social Research Council (ESRC), for example, or independent grant-making charities and trusts. Moreover, as long as certain academic standards are adhered to and maintained, these schemes give students and academics a unique opportunity to develop their own interests and ideas.

However, the opportunities for students and researchers to pursue and develop controversial and radical new ideas are limited, and, in my view, diminishing. Due mainly to the sustained critique of the social sciences by successive right-wing governments during the 1980s and early 90s, and the introduction of market forces into the university system, postgraduate training programmes are increasingly geared toward the acquisition of 'generic' rather than specific research skills. Also, established scholars with a good publication record are far more likely to get study leave or a research fellowship than their less illustrious colleagues with few or no publications. Furthermore, the recent erosion of job security within the university system, due mainly to the introduction of short-term contracts for new academic staff, can be seen as an implicit if not explicit incentive for anyone pursuing a career in academia to kow tow to convention.

Moreover, this situation has been exacerbated further by the Higher Education Funding Council's (HEFC) Research Assessment Exercise. Introduced in 1992 to bring the 'benefits' of market forces into the university system, and conducted every four years, the scheme grades university departments from one to five. High scoring departments receive significantly more funding from the HEFC than low scoring ones. Hence, those achieving a grade five, termed 'centres of excellence', have far more resources at their disposal than those deemed grade one or two. For academics, this can mean the difference between good working conditions and relative job security or possible redundancy. The two criteria used in the HEFC grading process are: the number and 'quality' of publications produced by individual academics working in a particular department and the amount of research they do. As a consequence, academic staff are 'encouraged' to produce at least four publications every 4 years, and to do as much research as possible.

The 'quality' of publications is judged by the level of 'scholarship' they exhibit. As a general rule, this means that complex and sophisticated analyses spread over hundreds of pages carry far more weight than relatively short single issue monographs and research reports. Articles published in 'academic' journals which are edited and refereed by academics, are rated far higher than those which appear in 'popular' magazines and newspapers like the Greater Manchester Coalition of Disabled People's *Coalition* or Scope's *Disability*

Now. Thus, the more sophisticated and, in most cases, the more inaccessible an academic's work is the more highly rated it is by the academic community.

In other words, the university system, implicitly if not explicitly, compels academics and researchers to write primarily for other academics and resarchers rather than for the general public. Or, to put it another way, and with regard to disability research, university based researchers are far more likely to write for other university based researchers than they are for their research subjects – disabled people.

Furthermore, postgraduate training programmes and research fellowships account for only a relatively small part of a research active university department's research activities. Most do research for external organisations on a subcontract basis. Additionally, the more money they can earn from research contracts, the higher their rating on the HEFC Research Assessment Exercise. With disability research this usually means policy related projects funded by health authorities, social services departments, charities and government departments.

For most of these organisations, disability remains a profoundly medical problem which warrants traditional individually based 'rehabilitative' type solutions that are both politically and professionally expedient. In many cases, these organisations are quite specific about their requirements and impose extensive constraints on what researchers can and cannot actually do. This is particularly evident with reference to government funded projects such as those initiated by the Department of Health (DH), National Health Service (NHS), and the Department of Employment (DE), for example.

Indeed, the main principle governing any Government funding of R&D (Research and Development) is the Rothschild principle, laid down in Cmd 4814 and reiterated in the White Paper 'Realising our potential: A Strategy for Science, Engineering and Technology', 'the customer says what he [*sic*] wants, the contractor does it, if he [*sic*] can and the customer pays' (DH, 1994a, p. 1).

According to the DH's code of practice, research and development commissioned by the Department should be commensurate with its policy and management aims. Furthermore, to ensure quality, research requirements must be informed by 'expert' advice, projects should follow a 'well defined protocol, be subjected to expert peer review, seek to maximise value for money, and meet agreed targets' (DH, 1994a, p. 1). A typical contract for DH funded research is about nine pages long and in several key areas is very explicit. Besides covering general arrangements for funding, administration and the staffing of projects they include instructions relating to research methodologies. For example, 'Any questionnaire, or forms used in surveys or both which are to form part of the research shall be submitted in draft to RDD (Research and Development Division) . . . together with explanatory notes, covering letters to respondents and any other relevant documents' (DH, 1994b, p. 4).

Additionally, if, for some reason, the DH is unhappy with how the research is being conducted then they have a legal right to terminate it as and when they feel appropriate. At the same time, if the research findings 'are vitiated by methodological problems . . . or otherwise'(?) (DH, 1994b, p. 7) then they are under no obligation to publish them.

It should also be remembered that the pressure on university based researchers to subscribe to this type of control is intensified by the commercialisation of social research. There are a number of research institutions, both large and small, which operate on a purely commercial basis tendering for lucrative research contracts.

Clearly, then, university based researchers are not free of external considerations and controls. To suggest otherwise is to misrepresent social research in the 1990s. Furthermore, in my view, to maintain the myth of the 'independent researcher' within the context of disability research – or any kind of social research, for that matter – can only exacerbate the gulf between researchers and research subjects – the very opposite of what is needed.

If disability research is about researching oppression, and I would argue that it is, then researchers should not be professing 'mythical independence' to disabled people, but joining with them in their struggles to confront and overcome this oppression. Researchers should be espousing commitment not value freedom, engagement not objectivity, and solidarity not independence. There is no independent haven or middle ground when researching oppression: academics and researchers can only be with the oppressors or with the oppressed.

References

Abberley, P. (1992) Counting us out: a discussion of the OPCS disability surveys, *Disability, Handicap and Society*, 7, pp. 139–157.

DH (1994a) *Department of Health Code of Practice for the Commissioning and Management of Research and Development* (London, Research and Development Division, Department of Health).

DH (1994b) *Specimen: conditions of approved cost contract* (London, Research and Development Division, Department of Health).

Hunt, P. (1981) Setting accounts with the parasite people, *Disability Challenge London, Union of the Physically Impaired Against Segregation*, No. 2, pp. 37–50.

Morris, J. (1992) Personal as political: a feminist perspective on researching physical disability, *Disability, Handicap and Society*, 7, pp. 157–166.

Oliver, M. (1990) *The Politics of Disablement* (London, Macmillan).

Oliver, M. (1992) Changing the social relations of research production, *Disability, Handicap and Society*, 7, pp. 101–115.

Pawson, R. (1989) *Measure for Measure: a manifesto for empirical sociology* (London, Routledge).

Rioux, M. and Bach, M. (1994) *Disability is Not Measles* (Ontario, L'Institut Roeher Institute).

Sayer, A. (1992) *Method in Social Science: a realist approach*, 2nd edn. (London, Routledge).

Part IV

Experiencing health and illness

Introduction

The growth in lay challenges to medicine's authority in health matters often centres on the inability of the medical profession to recognise and respond appropriately to the experience of health and illness which individuals and their families live through on a day-to-day basis. The experience of health and illness and the question of the relationship of this experience to underlying features of social structure such as social class is a major area of study in the sociology of health.

The existence of a wide variety of lay beliefs about health and illness, including lay theories of disease causation, has been shown to exist and is illustrated here by a short extract (Reading 24) from Blaxter's major study of 'health and lifestyles', in which four views of health are identified from a number of previous studies on lay concepts of health. These are health as absence of disease or illness, as the ability to function and perform one's social roles, as fitness, and finally as a reserve. Blaxter emphasises the complexity of lay concepts, that they often incorporate elements drawn from biomedicine as we have been encouraged to think in biomedical terms, and that 'people cannot always be expected to be consistent' in their view of health.

Variations in health belief influence the 'illness behaviour' which individuals engage in once they perceive that they have a health problem. The fact that health professionals only come into contact with the tip of an 'illness iceberg' is now well established. Consequently, seeking 'professional' advice or assistance is by no means a simple clear-cut process. Unlike the assumptions of functionalists such as Parsons who consider that, faced with illness, the (socially responsible) individual can be expected to consult medical opinion, sociologists working from an interactionist standpoint suggest that going to the doctor may well be a last resort once other avenues of advice and assistance have been exhausted. Zola's classic analysis (Reading 25) of the route from 'person' to 'patient' provides an excellent illustration of the complexities involved in 'illness behaviour'. According to Zola, the decision to go to the doctor is by no means as obvious a one as we might like to think, as for example following the appearance of clear objective symptoms where before there were none. Rather, Zola's study of a sample of patients new to outpatient clinics at Massachusetts General Hospital and seeking medical aid for the first time, suggests that individuals may have symptoms for a long time before seeking medical help, 'that there is an accommodation both physical, personal and social to the symptoms and it is when this accommodation breaks down that the person seeks, or is forced to seek medical aid'. What causes the accommodation to break down is the development of 'non-physiological patterns of triggers to the decision to seek medical aid'. From their data, Zola identifies five such patterns: interpersonal crisis, perceived interference with social or personal relations, sanctioning by a significant other, perceived interference with vocational or physical activity, and temporalising of symptoms. Significantly, these patterns of triggers are shown to be socially structured insofar as Zola concludes that the various ethnic groups in the study sample (Anglo-Saxon Protestant, Irish Catholic, Italian Catholic) 'favour particular decision-making patterns in the seeking of medical aid'.

The value of the interactionist perspective in the sociology of health, with its focus on micro encounters rather than macro structural analysis, has been significant. It has proved to be particularly fruitful in the analysis of face-to-face interaction between health professionals and patients. This is demonstrated in the Reader by an extract (Reading 26) from Stimson and Webb's study of the 'consultation process' between doctor and patient in a general practice setting. The medical consultation is viewed as a process of negotiation rather than as a predictable event whose outcome is simply dictated by the doctor's diagnosis of the patient's presenting problem. Both parties employ strategies, including their 'presentation of self', in their attempts to control the consultation and get the other party to accept their perspective on the situation. As each actor tries to influence the other, the actual outcome of the consultation will be the result of 'mutual interaction' between patient and doctor. Whilst emphasising the negotiable character of the face-to-face consultation, Stimson and Webb identify three 'limits' on the 'possibilities for action'. These are: (i) the way in which medical care is organised, which constrains the patient's access to a doctor; (ii) the patient's perception of 'what is possible', such as the amount of time available for consultation with the doctor; and (iii) 'areas of implicit agreement' which may restrict the scope for negotiation. Failure to identify such limitations as to what is negotiable can leave interactionists open to criticism that they neglect the impact of relations of 'power' and 'authority' in structuring encounters between health professionals and the lay population.

Interactionist accounts of professional/lay encounters in the health field do not, however, exhaust the theoretical perspectives brought to bear on the analysis of face-to-face interactions between health professionals and users of the health service. More recently, post-modern perspectives have shed new light on the processes of interaction, and in particular on the 'discursive conditions' which lend authority to medical discourse over lay discourse in such encounters. In this context see, for example, Nick Fox's recent analysis of surgeons' and patients' negotiations over discharge from hospital (Fox 1999).

Central to the experience of health and illness is the effects on lived experience of the 'social constructions' of health and illness which individuals variously face in their daily lives. Such constructions may significantly affect the 'quality' of living with an illness or the social response to individuals' 'health related behaviour', processes illustrated by two readings in the collection.

In the first (Reading 27), the experience of 'stigma' associated with certain illnesses is demonstrated in a discussion of the findings of a qualitative study which examined 'the experience of courtesy stigma among family members of persons with Alzheimer's disease'. 'Courtesy stigma' refers to the stigmatis-ation experienced by family members due to their close association with an individual who has a stigmatising illness. MacRae's findings confirm that it is common for relatives of individuals diagnosed with Alzheimer's disease to experience stigma and that this is not always confined to the primary caregiver but may extend to more distant relatives. The process of stigmatisation, however, is not simple, automatic or uniform, and its complexities are illus-trated by the fact that some family members successfully avoid becoming stigmatised if 'they are able to manipulate or control the definition of the situation so that others' reactions will not be negative'. A number of strategies employed by family members to manage or avoid stigma are identified and discussed, including 'medicalising the problem', concealing or covering up the illness, and utilising a 'technique of neutralisation' by which stigmatisation is avoided by refusing to accept and condone the negative reactions of others to the Alzheimer's sufferer. Central to this process of successfully negotiating a definition of the situation which allows 'courtesy stigma' to be avoided is 'the availability of "supportive others" who, although aware of the discreditable condition, are sympathetic and nonjudgemental' (p. 60).

Increasingly, individuals' and communities' 'health-related behaviour' is attracting political and social responses as cultural expectations of 'healthy lifestyles' and making 'healthy choices' become established as significant social norms. The response to 'unhealthy behaviour' is largely to regard it as socially deviant. That this common reaction fails to take account of the realities of unhealthy behaviour, including its health enhancing qualities, is powerfully illustrated by Hilary Graham's discussion of the lifestyles of a group of mothers on income support (Reading 28). Graham emphasises that the health-related behaviours of these women have to be understood in the context of the limited material and health resources with which they seek to care for their children. The health-damaging behaviours they engage in are then seen to be less of a lifestyle 'choice' than a 'compromise', a strategy to sustain the women in the face of daily routines which are heavily and unremittingly stressful. Cigarette smoking in particular is seen to provide these mothers with a rare break from their routines of caring and thereby exists as a means for both managing and defusing stress. In this respect it is experienced as 'a deeply contradictory habit' by these women, being both health-damaging in its consequences for the health of themselves and their children and existing as 'a child protective strategy, a resource which helped mothers cope with the demands of caring'. Graham's work offers a strong challenge to contemporary health policies which persist through their emphasis on individuals' managing their own lifestyles in focusing on individual behaviour removed from the social, cultural and material context which gives it sense.

As societies increasingly come to expect their citizens to manage their own health and take responsibility for their own illnesses, the individual is required to 'police their body'. In the sociology and politics of health, a sociology of the body has emerged as a rapidly expanding area following the impact of post-modernist theory. In the present collection, two readings focus on 'the body'. In the first (Reading 29), Featherstone examines the significance of the body to consumerism, and emphasises the important role that consumerist notions of the body have in 'health maintenance' and 'disease prevention' strategies and discourses. Within consumer culture the emphasis on 'appearance' and 'bodily presentation' has become paramount. The individual is encouraged to 'adopt instrumental strategies to combat deterioration and decay' with 'body work' being supported and structured through the production of 'stylised images of the body' in the advertising and entertainment media. In the context of consumer culture the prime purpose of individuals' maintaining their 'inner body' through control of their diet, exercise and unhealthy behaviours 'becomes the enhancement of the appearance of the outer body' (p. 18). Clearly, consumer culture is incapable of generating satisfactory strategies and solutions to the inevitable deterioration and decay which accompany ageing and death insofar as its logic is to avoid these realities and instead sell us the illusion of a forever happy, disease and pain-free life which we can achieve by buying into regimes of body maintenance.

Whilst buying into health and postponing ageing have become significant features of the experience of health and illness in late modernity, the need to tame and regulate our bodies has a much longer pedigree. The importance of body management to our everyday experience of social normality is illustrated by Seymour's recent examination of the issue of 'bodily continence' (Reading 30). Our preoccupation with bodily continence 'transcends age, gender, class and racial affiliation', and its social significance as an expression of adult citizenship is graphically illustrated in the case of adults whose specific health conditions render the routine maintenance of continence either difficult or impossible. Seymour draws on data from research conducted with a number of people experiencing 'varying degrees of bodily paralysis'. They describe what it is like to live in a 'leaking body' and their struggles to regain mastery over their bodies, a struggle which for many necessitates the suppression of spontaneity and freedom of choice which we all routinely exercise in relation to food and drink in return for a degree of bodily regulation. The accidental or traumatic nature of the event leading to bodily paralysis may be viewed as preventable and perceived to be in some way the result of individual irresponsibility. Under such circumstances, and in a culture which places such high value on individual's maintaining their health through the rational and responsible choices which they make, the person may feel under intense pressure to reaffirm control of their body as 'Successful body management, especially in the area of bodily continence, will provide evidence of a renewed sense of responsibility and commitment to core social values' (p. 160).

In the final contribution to the Reader (Reading 31), the question of the social nature of death and dying is addressed. For just as individuals' experience of health and illness is socially structured and constructed so the individual experience of dying is affected by cultural responses to death, responses which frame the possibility of achieving a 'good death'. McNamara's discussion identifies five 'inter-related' factors, which, it is argued, 'inform the manner in which people die in advanced industrial societies'. The factors and their cumulative effects confirm that far from being a simple biological fact, dying is a complex social process in which the unique experience of the terminally ill person is situated historically, socially and culturally.

References

Fox, N. (1999) ' "You can go home today Mrs Jones": surgeons' and patients' negotiations over discharge', in M. Purdy and D. Banks (eds) *Health and Exclusion: Policy and Practice in Health Provision*, London: Routledge.

24 Lay concepts of health*

Mildred Blaxter

What do people mean when they talk of 'health'? Since part of this analysis concerns people's attitudes to health, their ideas about the causes of illness, and the relationship between attitudes and behaviour, it is necessary to consider whether different people are thinking of health in entirely different ways. Clearly, concepts of health will affect ideas about responsibility.

Some researchers have gone so far as to suggest that, since health is essentially subjective, the only valid measure to accept is people's own assessment of whether they are healthy or not. There are, however, problems in adopting this approach, especially if we do not know what the respondents have in mind when they use the word 'health'. Standards vary among different social groups and depend very much on age and experience: self-assessments can be very individual and eccentric. Nevertheless, the outcome measures which are used in the analysis of a population survey ought at least to take some account of what health means to lay people.

A dichotomy has traditionally been seen between the biomedical or scientific model of health and a looser, more holistic model. These are sometimes falsely regarded as 'medical' and 'non-medical' ways of looking at health. Crudely, medical knowledge is seen as based on universal, generalizable science, and lay knowledge as unscientific, based on folk knowledge or individual experience. The lay concepts discussed in this chapter are not, however, being presented as necessarily or essentially different from medical concepts. In western societies, an intermixing is inevitable: lay people have been taught to think, at least in part, in bio-medical terms. Nor is modern medicine entirely wedded, in practice, to a narrowly-defined biomedical science: holistic concepts are also part of medical philosophy. The lay concepts which were expressed in this survey are, of course, sometimes less informed or expert than those of medical professionals. In other ways, however – since health must in part be sub-jectively experienced – they may be better informed. As other studies have found, they are often complex, subtle, and sophisticated.

*This is an extract from Blaxter, M. (1990) *Health and Lifestyles*, Routledge, pp. 13–16.

Previous studies of lay concepts

Lay concepts of health, among 'ordinary' people in western industrialized societies, have been seen as an interesting subject of research only during the past 15 years or so. Most studies have been relatively small in scale. Perhaps the most notable was one of the first: Herzlich's (1973) study of a sample of individuals, predominantly middle class, from Paris and Normandy. These respondents distinguished clearly between illness – the negative concept – which was produced by ways of life and especially urban life, and the positive concept of health, which came from within. Health was identified as having three dimensions: the simple absence of disease, a 'reserve' of health determined by temperament and constitution, and a positive state of well-being or 'equilibrium'.

Other studies, such as those of Pill and Stott (1982) among working-class mothers of young children in South Wales, Blaxter and Paterson (1982) among two generations of Scottish working-class women, Williams (1983) among elderly people in Scotland, or Blaxter (1985) among the patients of one general medical practice, have found rather similar distinctions. Health can be defined negatively, as the absence of illness, functionally, as the ability to cope with everyday activities, or positively, as fitness and well-being. It has also been noted that in the modern world, health still has a moral dimension. Ill health and moral wrong-doing can be connected, as much among industrialized and urban populations as among primitive societies: one has a duty to be healthy, and unhealthiness implies an element of failure. Health can be seen in terms of will-power, self-discipline and self-control (Blaxter 1983).

One problem about studies such as these is that they have concentrated on particular social groups, and it is difficult to know how generalizable the beliefs may be. Nevertheless, there have been several areas of agreement. The definition of health as positive fitness has been found to be more characteristic of those with better education or in more fortunate circumstances. In one large sample, in France, d'Houtard and Field (1984) found responses clearly linked to socio-economic class. The middle-class respondents were more likely to conceive of health in positive and expressive terms, the working class in negative and instrumental terms. Another, smaller, study of women in England (Calnan 1987) found a less clear-cut social class difference. Working-class women did, however, more frequently use an unidimensional definition that could be described as functional – 'the ability to get through the day' – while their professional counterparts were more likely to operate with multidimensional definitions which included the absence of illness and being fit as well as activity. It must be borne in mind, as Calnan points out, that these less elaborate answers of those with poorer education may be a product of the interview or survey situation, and cannot necessarily be presumed to represent differences in fundamental ideas. It has been shown in intensive, small-scale studies (Cornwell 1984, Blaxter 1983) that poorly-educated respondents, given time, can express very complex ideas on this topic. They do not always have them ready and fluent in a more superficial survey, however, and this may be relevant to the Health and Lifestyle Survey.

It is a general finding that, whatever their social class or education, people cannot always be expected to be consistent. It is very possible, as Williams (1983) has shown, to entertain two systems of thought on health-related topics at the same time, although they are at some point contradictory. These contradictions may be recognized by the informant, and elaborate attempts made to reconcile them.

Certainly, it is possible to define health as co-existing with quite severe disease or incapacity. Expressions of this from interview studies include, for instance, a Scottish woman who said of her husband that 'he had a lung taken out, but he was aye healthy enough' (Blaxter and Paterson 1982:28). Similarly, in another study, a daughter reported that her mother 'had been an active woman before this with no previous restriction apart from general old age, deafness, loss of sight in one eye and loss of memory. The doctor said at the inquest she was a very fit woman for her age' (Cartwright *et al.* 1973:41). Health or fitness have, in the minds of lay people, several different dimensions.

Alongside the three 'states' of health commonly identified – freedom from illness, ability to function, and fitness – the idea of health as 'reserve' has been found to be very prevalent. This reserve – like an economist's 'stock' of capital – can be diminished by self-neglect and accumulated by healthy behaviour. It is largely determined by heredity, influenced by childhood and traumatic events. Once spent, it leaves generalized weakness or vulnerability (Herzlich 1973; Pill and Stott 1982; Blaxter 1983). It can be exhausted, a state described by Williams' elderly respondents as being 'done, broken down, finished, cracked up, washed out', with some implication of irreversibility. Thus 'good' health is the power of overcoming disease, even if that disease is actually present: 'bad' health is being at risk, the loss of resistance even if disease is absent.

References

Blaxter, M. (1983) 'The causes of disease: women talking', *Social Science and Medicine* 17: 59–69.

Blaxter, M. (1985) 'Self-definition of health status and consulting rates in primary care', *Quarterly Journal of Social Affairs* 1: 131–71.

Blaxter, M. and Paterson, E. (1982) *Mothers and daughters: a three-generational study of health attitudes and behaviour*, London: Heinemann Educational Books.

Calnan, M. (1987) *Health and illness*, London: Tavistock.

Cartwright, A., Hockey, L., and Anderson, J.L. (1973) *Life before death*, London: Routledge & Kegan Paul.

Cornwell, J. (1984) *Hard-earned lives: accounts of health and illness from East London*, London: Tavistock Press.

d'Houtard, A. and Field, M.G. (1984) 'The image of health: variations in perception by social class in a French population', *Sociology of Health and Illness* 6: 30–60.

Herzlich, C. (1973) *Health and illness: a social psychological analysis*, London: Academic Press.

Pill, R. and Stott, N.C.H. (1982) 'Concept of illness causation and responsibility: some preliminary data from a sample of working class mothers', *Social Science and Medicine* 16: 43–52.

Williams, R.G.A. (1983) 'Concepts of health: an analysis of lay logic', *Sociology* 17: 185–204.

25 Pathways to the doctor – from person to patient*

Irving Kenneth Zola

The problem on which we wish to dwell is one about which we think we know a great deal but that, in reality, we know so little – how and why an individual seeks professional medical aid. The immediate and obvious answer is that a person goes to a doctor when he is sick. Yet, this term "sick", is much clearer to those who use it, namely the health practitioners and the researchers, than it is to those upon whom we apply it – the patients. Two examples may illustrate this point. Listen carefully to the words of a respondent in Koos' study of the Health of Regionville as she wrestled with a definition of this concept.

> "I wish I really knew what you meant about being sick. Sometimes I felt so bad I could curl up and die, but had to go on because the kids had to be taken care of and besides, we didn't have the money to spend for the doctor. How could I be sick? How do you know when you're sick, anyway? Some people can go to bed most anytime with anything, but most of us can't be sick, even when we need to be".[1]

Even when there is agreement as to what constitutes "sickness", there may be a difference of opinion as to what constitutes appropriate action, as in the following incident:

> A rather elderly woman arrived at the Medical Clinic of the Massachusetts General Hospital three days after an appointment. A somewhat exasperated nurse turned to her and said, "Mrs. Smith, your appointment was three days ago. Why weren't you here then?" To this Mrs. Smith responded, "How could I? Then I was sick."

Examples such as these are not unusual occurrences. And yet they cause little change in some basic working assumptions of the purveyors of medical care as well as the myriad investigators who are studying its delivery. It is to three of these assumptions we now turn: (1) the importance and frequency of

*This article was first published in *Social Science & Medicine*, vol. 7, pp. 677–89, 1973.

episodes of illness in an individual's life; (2) the representativeness of those episodes of illness which come to professional attention; and (3) the process by which an individual decides that a series of bodily discomforts he labels symptoms become worthy of professional attention. Together these assumptions create an interesting if misleading picture of illness. Rarely do we try to understand how or why a patient goes to the doctor, for the decision itself is thought to be an obvious one. We postulate a time when the patient is asymptomatic or unaware that he has symptoms, then suddenly some clear objective symptoms appear, then perhaps he goes through a period of self-treatment and when either this treatment is unsuccessful or the symptoms in some way become too difficult to take, he decides to go to some health practitioner (usually, we hope, a physician).

The first assumption, thus, deals with the idea that individuals at most times during their life are really asymptomatic. The extensive data pouring in from periodic health examination has gradually begun to question this notion. For, examinations of even supposedly healthy people, from business executives to union members to college professors, consistently reveal that at the time of their annual check-up, there was scarcely an individual who did not possess some symptom, some clinical entity worthy of treatment.[2] More general surveys have yielded similar findings.[3] Such data begins to give us a rather uncomfortable sense in which we may to some degree be sick every day of our lives. If we should even think of such a picture, however, the easiest way to dismiss this notion is that the majority of these everyday conditions are so minor as to be unworthy of medical treatment. This leads to our second assumption: namely, the degree of representativeness, both as to seriousness and frequency, of those episodes which do get to a doctor. Here too we are presented with puzzling facts. For if we look at investigations of either serious physical or mental disorder, there seem to be at least one, and in many cases several, people out of treatment for every person in treatment.[4] If, on the other hand, we look at a doctor's practice, we find that the vast bulk is concerned with quite minor disorders.[5] Furthermore, if we use symptom-check-lists or health calendars, we find that for these self-same minor disorders, there is little that distinguishes them medically from those that are ignored, tolerated, or self-medicated.[6]

With these confusions in mind, we can now turn to the third assumption. On the basis that symptoms were perceived to be an infrequent and thus somewhat dramatic event in one's life, the general assumption was that in the face of such symptoms, a rational individual after an appropriate amount of caution, would seek aid. When he does not or delays over-long, we begin to question his rationality. The innumerable studies of delay in cancer bear witness.

If we examine these studies we find that the reason for delay are a list of faults – the patient has no time, no money, no one to care for children, or take over other duties, is guilty, ashamed, fearful, anxious, embarrassed, or emotionally disturbed, dislikes physicians, nurses, hospitals, or needles, has had bad medical, familial or personal experiences, or is of lower education, socio-economic status, or an ethnic or racial minority.[7] As the researchers might put it, there is something about these people or in their backgrounds which has disturbed their rationality, for otherwise, they would "naturally" seek aid. And yet there is a curious methodological fact about these studies for all these investigations were done on *patients*, people who *had* ultimately decided to go to a physician. What happened? Were they no longer fearful? Did they get free time, more money, outside help? Did they resolve their guilt, shame, anxiety, distrust? No, this does not seem to have been the case. If anything the investigators seem to allude to the fact that the patients finally could not stand it any longer. Yet given the abundant data on the ability to tolerate pain[8] and a wide variety of other conditions, this notion of "not being able to stand it" simply does not ring true clinically.

We can now restate a more realistic empirical picture of illness episodes. Virtually every day of our lives we are subject to a vast array of bodily discomforts. Only an infinitesimal amount of these get to a physician. Neither the mere presence nor the obviousness of symptoms, neither their medical seriousness nor objective discomfort seems to differentiate those episodes which do and do not get professional treatment. In short, what then does convert a person to a patient? This then became a significant question and the search for an answer began.

At this point we had only the hunch that "something critical" must ordinarily happen to make an individual seek help. Given the voluminous literature on delay in seeking medical aid for almost every conceivable disorder and treatment, we might well say that that statistical norm for any population is to delay (perhaps infinitely for many). The implementing of this hunch is owed primarily to the intersection of two disciplines – anthropology and psychiatry. The first question to be faced was how and where to study this "something". Both prospective and retrospective studies were rejected. The former because as Professor H. M. Murphy noted there is often an enormous discrepancy between the declared intention and the actual act. The retrospective approach was rejected for two reasons – the almost notoriously poor recall that individuals have for past medical experiences and the distortions in recall introduced by the extensive "memory manipulation" which occurs as a result of the medical interview. Our resolution to this dilemma was a way of studying the patient when he was *in the process* of seeking medical aid. This process was somewhat artificially created by (1) interviewing patients while they waited to see their physician; (2) confining our sample to new patients to the Out-Patient Clinics of the Massachusetts General Hospital who were seeking aid for their particular problem for the first time. Thus, we had a group of people who were definitely committed to seeing a doctor (i.e. waiting) but who had not yet been subject to the biases and distortions that might occur through the medical interview (though some patients had been referred, we included only those on whom no definitive diagnosis had been made). This then was where we decided to study our problem.

In what to look for we were influenced by certain trends in general psychiatry away from defining mental illness solely in terms of symptoms possessed by a single isolated individual and instead conceptualizing it as a more general kind of disturbance in interpersonal behaviour and social living. (The resemblance that this bears to early classical notions of health and illness is quite striking. For then illness was conceived to be the disturbance between ego and his environment and not the physical symptom which happens to show up in ego).[9] On the empirical level we were influenced by the work of Clausen and his colleagues at the National Institute of Mental Health on the first admission to the hospital for male schizophrenics. Most striking about their material was the lack of any increase in the objective seriousness of the patient's disorder as a factor in this hospitalization. If anything, there was a kind of normalization in his family, an accommodation to the patient's symptoms. The hospitalization occurred not when the patient became sicker, but when the accommodation of the family, of the surrounding social context, broke down.[10] A translation of these findings could be made to physical illness. For, given all the data on delay, it seemed very likely that people have their symptoms for a long period of time before ever seeking medical aid. Thus one could hypothesize that there is an accommodation both physical, personal, and social to the symptoms and it is when this accommodation breaks down that the person seeks, or is forced to seek medical aid. Thus the "illness" for which one seeks help may only in part by a physical relief from symptoms. The research question on the decision to seek medical aid thus turned from the traditional focus on "why the delay" to the more general issue of "why come *now*". This way of asking this question is in itself not new. Physicians have often done it, but interestingly enough, they have asked it not in regard to general physical illness but rather when they can find nothing wrong. It is *then* that they feel that the patient may want or have been prompted to seek help for other than physical reasons.

The final issue which is essential to understanding the study concerns the nature of the sample. Here in particular there was an intersection of anthropology and psychiatry. Time and again anthropologists had called attention to the problem of designating certain behaviours as abnormal in one cultural situation but would be considered quite normal and even ignored in another. Usually, when they explained this phenomenon they did so in terms of value-orientations; namely that there was something about the fit or lack of fit of the particular problem (symptom or sign), into a larger cultural pattern which helped explain why it was or was not abnormal.[11] Why could not the same process be operating in regard to physical symptoms? Perhaps many of the unexplained epidemiological differences between groups may also be due to the fact that in one group the particular physical sign is considered normal and in the second group not. For given the enormous tolerance we have for many physical conditions, given that our morbidity statistics are based primarily on treated disorders, many of these differences may reflect differences in attention and not differences in prevalence or incidence. While anthropologists have reported their findings mostly in comparisons of non-literate groups with a more "modern" society, we decided to translate their idea of a culture into a contemporary format. We thus speculated that ethnic groups, particularly in an area such as Boston, Massachusetts, might well function as cultural reference groups and thus be an urban transmitter and perpetuator of value-orientations. The specific ethnic groups we studied were determined by a demographic study at the Massachusetts General Hospital, from which we were able to determine the three most populous ethnic groups, Italian, Irish Catholic and Anglo-Saxon Protestant.

To summarize the methodological introduction, in our first study, the sample consisted of patients completely new to the out-patient clinics who were seeking medical aid for the first time for this particular problem, who were between the ages of 18 and 50, able to converse in English, of either Anglo-Saxon Protestant, Irish Catholic or Italian Catholic background. The data-collection took place at the three clinics to which these groups were most frequently sent – the Eye Clinic, the Ear, Nose and Throat Clinic, and the Medical Clinic, which were, incidentally, three of the largest clinics in the hospital. The interviewing took place during the waiting time before they saw their physicians with the general focus of the questioning being: Why did you seek medical aid now? In addition to many such open-ended questions, we had other information derived from the medical record, demographic interviews, attitude scales and check lists. We also had each examining physician fill out a medical rating sheet on each patient. In all we saw over two hundred patients, fairly evenly divided between male and female.[12]

We first examined the presenting complaints of the patients to see if there were differing conceptions of what is symptomatic.[13] Our first finding dealt with the location of their troubles. The Irish tended to place the locus of symptoms in the eye, the ear, the nose or the throat – a sense organ while the Italians showed no particular clustering. The same result obtained when we asked what was the most important part of the body. Here too the Irish tended to place their symptoms in the eyes, ears, nose and throat with the Italians not favouring any specific location. We noted, however, that this was not merely a reflection of epidemiological differences; for Italians who did have eye, ear, nose and throat problems did not necessarily locate their chief complaint in either the eye, ear, nose or throat. We thus began to wonder if this focussing was telling us something other than a specific location. And so we turned our attention to more qualitative aspects of symptoms, such as the presence of pain. Here we noted that the Italians much more often felt that pain constituted a major part of their problem, whereas the Irish felt equally strongly that it did not. However, we had our first clue that "something else" was going on. The Irish did not merely say they had no pain, but rather utilized a kind of denial with such statements as, "No, I wouldn't call it a pain, rather a discomfort"; or "No, a slight headache, but nothing that lasts". Further analysis of our data then led us to create a typology in which we tried to grasp the essence of a patient's complaint. One type seemed to reflect a rather specific organic dysfunctioning (difficulty in seeing, inappropriate functioning, discharge, or movement etc.) while the second type represented a more global malfunctioning (aches and pains, appearance, energy level etc). Looked at in this way, we found that significantly more Irish seemed to describe their problem in terms of a rather specific dysfunction whereas the Italians described their complaints in a more diffuse way. Thus, the Irish seemed to convey a concern with something specific, something that has gone wrong, or been impaired; whereas the Italian is concerned with or conveyed a more global malfunctioning emphasizing the more diffuse nature of their complaints.

We now had differentiated two ways of communicating about one's bodily complaints – a kind of restricting versus generalizing tendency and we thus sought evidence to either refute or substantiate it. Two "tests" suggested themselves. The first consisted of three sets of tabulations: (1) the total number of symptoms a patient had; (2) the total number of different types of malfunctions from which he suffered (the typology mentioned above actually consisted of nine codifiable categories); and (3) the total number of different parts of the body in which a patient located complaints. Each we regarded as a measure of "generalizing" one's complaints. As we predicted the Italians had significantly more complaints of a greater variety, and in more places than did the Irish. Our second "test" consisted of several questions dealing with the effect of their symptoms on their interpersonal behaviour. Here we reasoned that the Irish would be much more likely to restrict the effect of their symptoms to physical functioning. And so it was, with the Italians claiming that the symptoms interfered with their general mode of living and the Irish just as vehemently denying any such interference. Here again, the Irish presented a "no with a difference" in such statements as "No, there may have been times that I become uncomfortable physically and afraid to show it socially. If I felt that way I even tried to be a little more sociable."

Perhaps the best way to convey how differently these two groups communicated their symptoms is by a composite picture [Table 1]. The two series of responses were given by an Italian and an Irish patient of similar age and sex, with a disorder of approximately the same duration and seriousness and with the same primary and, if present, secondary diagnosis.

The crux of the study is, however, the decision to see a doctor. One of our basic claims was that the decision to seek medical aid was based on a break in the accommodation to the symptoms, that in the vast majority of situations, an individual did not seek aid at his physically sickest point. We do not mean by this that symptoms were unimportant. What we mean is that they function as a sort of constant and that when the decision to seek medical aid was made the physical symptoms alone were not sufficient to prompt this seeking. Typical of the amount of debilitation people can tolerate as well as the considerable seriousness and still the decision to seek medical attention made on extra-physical grounds is the case of Mary O'Rourke.

Table 1

Diagnosis	Question of interviewer	Irish patient	Italian patient
1. Presbyopia and Hyperopia	What seems to be the trouble?	I can't see to thread a needle or read a paper.	I have a constant headache and my eyes seem to get all red and burny
	Anything else?	No, I can't recall any.	No, just that it lasts all day long and I even wake up with it sometimes.
2. Myopia	What seems to be the trouble?	I can't see across the street.	My eyes seem very burny, especially the right eye . . . Two or three months ago I woke up with my eye swollen. I bathed it and it did go away but there was still the burny sensation.
	Anything else?	I have been experiencing headaches but it may be that I'm in early menopause.	Yes, there always seems to be a red spot beneath this eye . . .
	Anything else?	No.	Well, my eyes feel very heavy . . . at night they bother me most.

These cases have been chosen precisely because they are relatively minor disorders. So straightforward are they that one should expect very little difference between patients who are their "owners". And yet not only does the Italian patient consistently present more troubles than the Irish but while the Irish patient focussed on a specific malfunctioning as the main concern, the Italian did not even mention this aspect of the problem but focussed on more "painful" and diffuse qualities of his condition.

Mary O'Rourke is 49, married and is a licensed practical nurse. Her symptom was a simple one, "The sight is no good in this eye . . . can't see print at all, no matter how big". This she claimed was due to being hit on the side of the head by a baseball 4 months ago, but she just couldn't get around to a doctor before this. Why did she decide now, did her vision become worse? "Well . . . about a month ago I was taking care of his (a client's) mother . . . he mentioned that my eyelid was drooping . . . it was the first time he ever did . . . if he hadn't pointed it out I wouldn't have gone then". "Why did you pay attention to his advice?" "Well it takes away from my appearance . . . bad enough to feel this way without having to look that way . . . the same day I told my husband to call." Diagnosis – Chorioretinitis O.S. (permanent partial blindness) "lesion present much

longer than present symptoms". Incidentally, no "drooping" was noticeable to either the interviewer or the examining physician.

Case after case could be presented to make this point but even more
striking is that there is a "method underlying this madness". In our data we
were able to discern several distinct non physiological patterns of triggers to
the decision to seek medical aid. We have called them as follows: (1) the
occurrence of an interpersonal crisis; (2) the *perceived* interference with social
or personal relations; (3) sanctioning; (4) the *perceived* interference with
vocational or physical activity; and (5) a kind of temporalizing of symptomatology. Moreover, these five patterns were clustered in such a way that we
could characterize each ethnic group in our sample as favouring particular
decision-making patterns in the seeking of medical aid.

The first two patterns, the presence of an interpersonal crisis, and the
perceived interference with social or personal relations were more frequent
among the Italians. The former, that of a crisis, does not mean that the
symptoms have led to a crisis or even vice-versa, but that the crisis called
attention to the symptoms, caused the patient to dwell on them and finally to
do something about them. Two examples will illustrate this.

Jennie Bella was 40, single, and had a hearing difficulty for many years.
She said that the symptoms have not gotten worse nor do they bother her
a great deal (Diagnosis: Non-supporative Otitis Media) and, furthermore,
she admitted being petrified of doctors. "I don't like to come . . . I don't
like doctors. I never did . . . I have to be unconscious to go . . . ." She can
nevertheless not pinpoint any reason for coming at this time other than
a general feeling that it should be taken care of. But when she was
questioned about her family's concern, she blurted out, "I'm very
nervous with my mother, up to this year I've been quiet, a stay-at-home
. . . Now I've decided to go out and have some fun. My mother is very
strict and very religious. She doesn't like the idea of my going out with a
lot of men. She don't think I should go out with one for awhile and then
stop. She says I'm not a nice girl, that I shouldn't go with a man unless I
plan to marry . . . she doesn't like my keeping late hours or coming home
late. She always suspects the worst of me . . . This year it's just been
miserable . . . I can't talk to her . . . she makes me very upset and its been
getting worse . . . The other day . . . last week we (in lowered tones) had
the argument." Miss Bella called for an appointment the next morning.

Carol Conte was a 45-year-old, single, bookkeeper. For a number of
years she had been both the sole support and nurse for her mother.
Within the past year, her mother died and shortly thereafter her relatives
began insisting that she move in with them, quit her job, work in their
variety store and nurse their mother. With Carol's vacation approaching,
they have stepped up their efforts to persuade her to at least try this

arrangement. Although she has long had a number of minor aches and pains, her chief complaint was a small cyst on her eyelid (Diagnosis: Fibroma). She related her fear that it *might* be growing or could lead to something more serious and thus she felt she had better look into it now (the second day of her vacation) "before it was too late". "Too late" for what was revealed only in a somewhat mumbled response to the question of what she expected or would like the doctor to do. From a list of possible outcomes to her examination, she responded, "Maybe a 'hospital' (isation) . . . 'Rest' would be all right . . . (and then in a barely audible tone, in fact turning her head away as if she were speaking to no one at all) "just so they (the family) would stop bothering me." Responding to her physical concern, the examining physician acceded to her request for the removal of the fibroma, referred her for surgery and thus removed her from the situation for the duration of her vacation.

In such cases, it appeared that regardless of the reality and seriousness of the symptoms, they provide but the rationale for an escape, the calling-card or ticket to a potential source of help – the doctor.

The second pattern – the perceived interference with social or personal relations – is illustrated by the following two Italian patients.

John Pell is 18 and in his senior year of high school. For almost a year he's had headaches over his left eye and pain in and around his right, artificial, eye. The symptoms seem to be most prominent in the early evening. He claimed, however, little general difficulty or interference until he was asked whether the symptoms affected how he got along. To this he replied, "That's what worries me . . . I like to go out and meet people and now I've been avoiding people". Since he has had this problem for a year, he was probed as to why it bothered him more at this particular time. "The last few days of school it bothered me so that I tried to avoid everybody (this incidentally was his characteristic pattern *whenever* his eyes bothered him) . . . and I want to go out with . . . and my Senior Prom coming up, and I get the pains at 7 or 7.30 how can I stay out . . . then I saw the nurse." To be specific, he was walking down the school corridor and saw the announcement of the upcoming Prom. He noticed the starting time of 8 p.m. and went immediately to the school nurse who in turn referred him to the Massachusetts Eye and Ear Infirmary.

Harry Gallo is 41, married, and a "trainee" at a car dealers. "For a very long time my trouble is I can't drink . . . tea, coffee, booze . . . eat ice cream, fried foods. What happens is I get pains if I do have it." (Diagnosis: peptic ulcer). He becomes very dramatic when talking about how the symptoms affected him. "It shot my social life all to pieces . . . we all want to socialize . . . and it's a tough thing. I want to go with people, but I can't. Wherever we go they want to eat or there's food and

I get hungry . . . and if I eat there, I get sick." Of course, he has gone off his "diet" and has gotten sick. Most of the time he watches himself and drinks Malox. He saw a doctor once 2 years ago and has been considering going again but, "I kept putting it off . . . because I got lazy . . . there were so many things. I've just been starting a new job and I didn't want to start taking off and not working, but this last attack was *too much*!" He then told how day after day the "boys at work" have been urging him to stop off with them for a few quick ones. He knew he shouldn't but he so wanted to fit in and so "It was with the boys and the other salesmen . . . I drank beer . . . I knew I was going to have more than one . . . and . . . *it* happened on the way home. . . ." Storming into his home, he asked his wife to make an appointment at the hospital, stating almost exasperatingly, "if you can't drink beer with friends, what the hell . . .".

In these cases, the symptoms were relatively chronic. At the time of the decision there may have been an acute episode, but this was not the first such time the symptoms had reached such a "state" but rather it was the perception of them on this occasion as interfering with the social and interpersonal relations that was the trigger or final straw.

The third pattern, sanctioning, was the overwhelming favourite of the Irish. It is, however, not as well illustrated by dramatic examples, for it consists simply of one individual taking the primary responsibility for the decision to seek aid for someone else. For many weeks it looked as if one were seeing the submissive half of a dominant–submissive relationship. But within a period of 6 months, a husband and wife appeared at the clinics and each one assumed the role of sanctioning for the other.

Mr. and Mrs. O'Brien were both suffering from Myopia, both claimed difficulty in seeing, both had had their trouble for some period of time. The wife described her visit as follows: "Oh, as far as the symptoms were concerned, I'd be apt to let it go, but not my husband. He worries a lot, he wants things to be just so. Finally when my brother was better he (the husband) said to me: "Your worries about your brother are over so why can't you take care of your eyes now?" And so she did. Her husband, coming in several months later, followed the same pattern. He also considered himself somewhat resistant to being doctored. "I'm not in the habit of talking about aches and pains. My wife perhaps would say 'Go to the doctor', but me, I'd like to see if things will work themselves out." How did he get here? It turns out that he was on vacation and he'd been meaning to take care of it, "Well I tend to let things go but not my wife, so on the first day of my vacation my wife said, 'Why don't you come, why don't you take care of it now?' So I did."

Thus in these cases both claimed a resistance to seeing a doctor, both claimed the other is more likely to take care of such problems, and yet both served as the pushing force to the other. Interestingly enough, the dramatic aspect of such cases was not shown in those who followed the general pattern which was often fairly straightforward, but in those cases which did not. Two examples illustrate this. One was a woman with a thyroid condition, swelling on the side of the neck who when asked why she came at this time blurted out almost in a shout, "Why did I come now? I've been walking around the house like this for several weeks now and nobody said anything so I *had to come myself*". Or the almost plaintive complaint of a veteran, kind of grumbling when asked why he came now, begrudged the fact that he had to make a decision himself with the statement, "Hmm, in the Navy they just take you to the doctor, you don't have to go yourself". It is not that these people are in any sense stoic, for it seemed that they were quite verbal and open about complaining but just that they did not want to take the responsibility on themselves.

There is a secondary pattern of the Irish, which turns out to be also the major pattern of the Anglo-Saxon group.[14] It was almost straight out of the Protestant ethic: namely a perceived interference with work or physical functioning. The word "perceived" is to be emphasized because the nature of the circumstances range from a single woman, 35 years old, who for the first time noted that the material which she was typing appeared blurred and thus felt that she had better take care of it, to a man with Multiple Sclerosis who despite falling down and losing his balance in many places, did nothing about it until he fell at work. Then he perceived that it might have some effect on his work and his ability to continue. The secondary Anglo-Saxon pattern is worth commenting on, for at first glance it appears to be one of the most rational modes of decision-making. It is one that most readers of this paper may well have used, namely the setting of external time criteria. "If it isn't better in 3 days, or 1 week, or 7 hours, or 6 months, then I'll take care of it." A variant on this theme involves the setting of a different kind of temporal standard – the recurrence of the phenomenon. A 19-year-old college sophomore reported the following:

> "Well, it was this way. I went into this classroom and sat in the back of the room and when the professor started to write on the blackboard I noticed that the words were somewhat blurry. But I didn't think too much about it. A couple of weeks later, when I went back into the same classroom, I noted that it was blurry again. Well, once was bad, but twice that was too much."

Now given that his diagnosis was Myopia and that it was unconnected with any other disease, we know medically that his Myopia did not vary from one circumstance to another. This imposition of "a first time, second time that's too much" was of his doing and unrelated to any medical or physical reality.

By now the role that symptoms played in the decision to seek medical aid should be clearer. For our patients the symptoms were "really" there, but their perception differed considerably. There *is* a sense in which they sought help because they could not stand it any longer. But what they could not stand was more likely to be a situation or a perceived implication of a symptom rather than any worsening of the symptom *per se*.

I now would like to note some of the implications of this work. When speaking of implications, I ask your indulgence, for I refer not merely to what leads in a direct line from the data but some of the different thoughts and directions in which it leads me. What for example are the consequences for our very conception of etiology – conceptions based on assumptions about the representativeness of whom and what we study. We have claimed in this paper that the reason people get into medical treatment may well be related to some select social psychological circumstances. If this is true, it makes all the more meaningful our earlier point about many unexplained epidemiological differences, for they may be due more to the differential occurrence of these social-psychological factors, factors of selectivity and attention which get people and their episodes into medical statistics rather than to any true difference in the prevalence and incidence of a particular problem or disorder.[15] Our findings may also have implications for what one studies, particularly to the importance of stress in the etiology of so many complaints and disorders. For it may well be that the stress noted in these people's lives, at least those which they were able to verbalize, is the stress which brought them into the hospital or into seeking treatment (as was one of our main triggers) and not really a factor in the etiology or the exacerbation of the disorder.

Our work also has implications for treatment. So often we hear the terms "unmotivated, unreachable and resistance" applied to difficult cases. Yet we fail to realize that these terms may equally apply to us, the caretakers and health professionals who may not understand what the patient is saying or if we do, do not want to hear it. An example of this was seen in the way physicians in this study handled those patients for whose problem no organic basis could be found.[16] For despite the fact that there were no objective differences in the prevalence of emotional problems between our ethnic groups, the Italians were consistently diagnosed as having some psychological difficulty such as tension headaches, functional problems, personality disorder, etc; whereas the Irish and Anglo-Saxon were consistently given what one might call a neutral diagnosis, something that was either a Latinized term for their symptoms or simply the words "nothing found on tests" or "nothing wrong". Our explanation is somewhat as follows, namely that this situation is one of the most difficult for a physician and one in which he nevertheless feels he should make a differential diagnosis. Faced with this dilemma he focussed inordinately on *how* the Italians presented themselves – somewhat voluble, with many more symptoms, and somewhat dramatic social circumstances surrounding their decision to seek help. This labelling of the Italians is particularly interesting since as we mentioned above the Irish and Anglo-Saxons had similar psychological and social problems but presented them in a much more emotionally neutral and bland manner. There are no doubt other factors operating such as the greater social distance between the Italians and the medical staff but that would constitute another paper.

One final remark as to treatment, again and again we found that where the physician paid little attention to the specific trigger which forced or which the individual used as an excuse to seek medical aid, there was the greatest likelihood of that patient eventually breaking off treatment. Another way of putting this is that without attention to this phenomenon the physician would have no opportunity to practise his healing art. Moreover, this problem of triggers etc. brooked no speciality nor particular type of disorder. So that being a specialist and only seeing certain kinds of problems did not exempt the physician from having to deal with this issue.

Such data alone supports those who urge more training in social and psychological sophistication for *any* physician who has contact with patients. With chronic illness making up the bulk of today's health problems it is obvious that the physicians cannot treat the etiological agent of disease and that the effect of specific therapies is rather limited. Nevertheless the physician may more intelligently intervene in the patient's efforts to cope with his disorder if he has the knowledge and awareness of the patient's views of health, sickness, his expectations and his reasons for seeking help.

This report has several different goals. To the social scientist we have tried to convey the somewhat amazing persistence of certain cultural characteristics which we in our cultural blindness have felt should have died and disappeared. The reason for their survival is that such behaviours may well be general modes of handling anxiety, sort of culturally prescribed defence mechanisms and probably transmitted from generation to generation in the way that much learning takes place, almost on an unconscious level. If this be true, then they constitute a group of behaviours which are much less likely to be changed as one wishes or attempts to become more American. Hopefully, the present research has also demonstrated the fruitfulness of an approach which does not take the definition of abnormality for granted. Despite its limitations our data seems sufficiently striking to invite further reason for re-examining our traditional and often rigid conceptions of health and illness, of normality and abnormality, of conformity and deviance. As we have contended in the early pages of this essay, symptoms or physical aberations are so widespread that perhaps relatively few, and a biased selection at best, come to the attention of official treatment agencies. We have thus tried to present evidence showing that the very labelling and definition of a bodily state as a symptom as well as the decision to do something about it is in itself part of a social process. If there is a selection and definitional process then focussing solely on reasons for deviation (the study of etiology) and the reasons for not seeking treatment (the study of delay) and ignoring what constitutes a deviation in the eyes of an individual and his reasons for action may obscure important aspects of our understanding and eventually our philosophy of the treatment and control of illness.

Finally, this is not meant to be an essay on the importance of sociological factors in disease, but rather the presentation of an approach to the study of health and illness. Rather than being a narrow and limited concept, health and illness are on the contrary empirically quite elastic. In short, it is not merely that health and illness has sociological aspects, for it has many aspects, but really that there is a sense in which health and illness *are* social phenomena. The implication of this perspective has perhaps been much better put by the Leightons (though quoted out of context):

> "From this broad perspective there is no point in asking whether over the span of his adult life a particular individual should or should not be considered a medical case – everyone is a medical case. The significant question becomes how severe a case, what kind of case."[17]

I myself would add – how does one become a case and since of the many eligible, so few are chosen, what does it mean to be a case. In an era where every day produces new medical discoveries, such questions are all too easily ignored. The cure for all men's ills seems right over the next hill. Yet as Dubos has cogently reminded us,[18] this vision is only a mirage and the sooner we realize it the better.

References

1 Koos, Earl L. *The Health of Regionville*, Columbia University Press, New York, 1954.
2 General summaries: Meigs, J. Wistar. Occupational medicine. *New Eng. J. Med.* **264**, 861, 1961; Siegel, Gordon S. *Periodic Health Examinations – Abstracts from the Literature*, Public Health Service Publication, No. 1010, U.S. Government Printing Office, Washington D.C., 1963.
3 See for example: Commission on Chronic Illness, *Chronic Illness in a Large City*, Harvard University Press, Cambridge, 1957; Pearse, Innes H. and Crocker, Lucy H. *The Peckham Experiment*, Allen & Unwin, London, 1954; *Biologists in Search of Material*, Interim Reports of the Work of the Pioneer Health Center, Faber & Faber, London, 1938.
4 Commission on Chronic Illness, *op. cit.*; Pearse and Crocker, *op. cit.*.
5 Clute, Y. T. *The General Practitioner*, University of Toronto Press, Toronto, 1963, as well as many of the articles cited in Stoekle, John D., Zola, Irving K. and Davidson, Gerald E. The quantity and significance of psychological distress in medical patients. *J. Chron. Dis.*, **17**, 959, 1964.
6 Unpublished data of the author and also Kosa, John, Alpert, Joel, Pickering, M. Ruth and Haggerty, Robert J. Crisis and family life: a re-examination of concepts. *The Wisconsin Sociologist* **4**, 11, 1965; Kosa, John, Alpert, Joel and Haggerty, Robert J. On the reliability of family health information. *Soc. Sci & Med.* **1**, 165, 1967; Alpert, Joel, Kosa John and Haggerty, Robert J. A month of illness and health care among low-income families. *Publ. Hlth. Rep.* **82**, 705, 1967.
7 Blackwell, Barbara. The literature of delay in seeking medical care for chronic illnesses. *Hlth Educ. Monographs* No. 16, pp. 3–32, 1963; Kutner, Bernard, Makover, Henry B. and Oppenheim, Abraham. Delay in the diagnosis and treatment of cancer.

J. Chron. Dis. **7**, 95, 1958; Kutner, Bernard and Gordon, Gerald. Seeking aid for cancer. *J. Hlth Hum. Behav.* **2**, 171, 1961.

8 Chapman, William P. and Jones, Chester M. Variations in cutaneous and visceral pain sensitivity in normal subjects. *J. Clin. Invest.* **23**, 81, 1944; Hardy, James D., Wolff, Harold G. and Goodell, Helen. *Pain Sensations and Reactions* Williams & Wilkins, Baltimore, 1952; Melzack, Ronald. The perception of pain. *Scient. Am.* **204**, 41, 1961; Olin, Harry S. and Hackett, Thomas P. The denial of chest pain in 32 patients with acute myocardial infection. *J. Am. Med. Ass.* **190**, 977, 1964.

9 Galdston, Iago. (editor) Salerno and the atom. In *Medicine in a Changing Society*, pp. 111–161. International Universities Press, New York, 1956.

10 Clausen, John A. and Radke Yarrow, Marian. The impact of mental illness on the family. *J. Soc. Iss.* **11**, 1, 1955.

11 Opler, Marvin K. *Culture, Psychiatry and Human Values*, Charles C. Thomas, Springfield, Illinois, 1956; Opler, Marvin K. (editor) *Culture and Mental Health*, MacMillan, New York, 1959.

12 All differences reported here are statistically significant. Given that there are no tabular presentations in this essay it may be helpful to remember that for the most part we are not stating that all or necessarily a majority of a particular group acted in the way depicted but that at the very least, the response was significantly more peculiar to this group than to any other. Moreover, all the reported differences were sustained even when the diagnosed disorder for which they sought aid was held constant. For details on some of the statistical procedures as well as some of the methodological controls, see Zola, Irving K. Culture and symptoms – an analysis of patients' presenting complaints. *Am. Sociol. Rev.* **31**, 615, 1966.

13 The findings re. symptoms are primarily a contrast between the Irish and the Italians. This is done because (1) there is a sense in which ethnicity in Boston is a much more "real" phenomenon to the Irish and the Italians than to our Anglo-Saxon Protestant, (2) these two groups are more purely "ethnic" and constitute a fairer comparison being of similar generation, education, and socio-economic status, and (3) the differences are frankly much more dramatic and clearly drawn. If you wish to picture where the Anglo-Saxons might be in these comparisons, think of them as mid-way between the Irish and Italian responses, if anything, a little closer to the Irish. Some further discussion of this issue is found both in Zola, Irving K., Culture and symptoms, *op. cit.*, and Illness behaviour in the working class. In *Blue Collar World* (edited by Shustak, Arthur B. and Gomberg, William) pp. 350–361. Prentice Hall, Englewood Cliffs, N.J., 1964.

14 As we have argued elsewhere (Zola, Irving K. Illness behavior . . ., *op. cit.*) this and the following pattern are also characteristic of more middle-class and more highly educated groups.

15 Mechanic, David and Volkart, Edmund H. Illness behavior and medical diagnosis. *J. Hlth Hum. Behav.* **1**, 86, 1960.

16 Detailed in Zola, Irving K. Problems of communication, diagnosis and patient care: the interplay of patient physician and clinic organization. *J. Med. Educ.* **38**, 829, 1963.

17 Leighton, Dorothea C., Harding, John S., Macklin, David B., MacMillam, Allister H. and Leighton, Alexander H. *The Character of Danger*, pp. 135–136. Basic Books, New York, 1963.

18 Dubos, Rene. *Mirage of Health*, Anchor, Garden City, New York, 1961; Dubos, Rene. *Man Adapting*, Yale, New Haven, Conn., 1965.

26 Going to see the doctor*

Gerry Stimson and Barbara Webb

The face-to-face interaction

> The study of the patient perspective must be undertaken within the assumption that he is as much a participant in the play as he is recipient or audience.
>
> Hans O. Mauksch, 1972, p. 27

Two themes guide our analysis of the face-to-face consultation: strategies and negotiation. Essentially both actors (although we concentrate on the patient) are concerned with the same problem. This problem is effective self-presentation. As in all interaction, the conscious and unconscious presentation of the self affects the behaviour of the other and calls forth a reaction by the other. But in the consultation there is the problem of the outcome that is desired by both actors. People do not hand over all control and decision-making to the doctor merely by becoming patients. The presentation of the self can be used as a strategy. The aim of the strategies used by both patient and doctor is to attempt to control and direct the consultation along their own desired lines, to persuade the other to recognise or accept a particular perspective on, and orientation to, the problem that has been brought.

Seeing the consultation in terms of each actor trying to influence the other brings in the concept of negotiation. For, far from the outcome of the consultation being determined only by the problem that the patient brings and by the diagnosis of the doctor, the outcome is a result of the mutual interaction. An examination of the literature on the diagnostic process (Maddox, 1973) suggests that there is so much room for variability in diagnosis, even with seemingly 'hard' information such as the results of X-ray photographs, that diagnosis is not the cut-and-dried scientific exercise that it is often made out to be. Roth (1963) discusses this problem of diagnosis and treatment in his study of the career of the patient with tuberculosis. Patients and doctors argue about the interpretation of tests, about what treatment is necessary, about the pacing of treatment and about restrictions on their

*This is an extract from Stimson, G. and Webb, B. (1975) *Going to See the Doctor: The Consultation Process in General Practice*, Routledge & Kegan Paul, pp. 37–41.

behaviour at different stages in the treatment. Roth sees the treatment of the tuberculosis patient not as the result of specific treatment plans and decisions made by the medical staff but as emerging from the ongoing negotiation and bargaining between the patient and the medical staff.

In the psychiatric interview, Scheff (1968) has shown how the reality of the patient's problem is negotiated by the psychiatrist. In the example of the psychiatric interview which he gives, an interview which is taken from a gramophone record for teaching psychiatrists, the psychiatrist is faced with a woman who comes to him with a problem which she at first blames on her husband. By the end of the interview the psychiatrist has the patient agreeing that the problem might lie more in herself than in her husband. In a study of doctor–patient interactions in two paediatric out-patient clinics Strong and Davis (1972) describe how parents have their own definitions of their child's problem: 'Both doctor and patient can accept or reject the other's categorisations . . . The diagnostic outcome of the interview is therefore continually negotiated.' The doctor is shown as using various techniques to maintain his status as expert, particularly when faced by the parents' 'loss of faith' in his competence.

Negotiation is a process. That patient and doctor both use strategies to influence each other does not mean that one or other is going to be successful. But the concept of negotiation means that we see the outcome as the result of their interaction and the strategies they have each adopted, rather than as determined solely by the facts that are brought and the application of the skills that the doctor has.

The consultation does not take place in a vacuum. First, both doctor and patient may have met before and will have foreknowledge of each other. This, as we have seen, allows the patient to anticipate the consultation and rehearse strategies. Where the doctor and illness condition are well known and the patient feels certain of the encounter and able to predict its probable course, we suggest that presentation and control strategies may have less of a persuasive content and the effort may be concentrated on reinforcing a common understanding and on following the usual pattern of activity. The most obvious example of this is the repeat prescription régime, which Marinker (1970) refers to as the 'truce', where a pattern of consultation has become routine. Yet negotiation does not cease; the inference behind the stereotyped actions is that reinforcement is necessary in order to ensure the continuation of such relations. Of course it may happen that the approach of the doctor is well known but the patient is dissatisfied with that approach. For example, a doctor may tend to treat many conditions with his 'favourite drug' and the patient may desire some other form of treatment. Or he may be predisposed to certain actions:

> '[He is known as] Doctor Undress – he makes you strip to the waist and that's only when you've got a sore throat, and he is very partial to internals for everything you have.'

The patient may feel this behaviour is inappropriate and tactics may then be used by the patient to dissuade the doctor from his usual routine. Although strategies such as these may be planned through the patient having prior expectations of the encounter and having anticipated the problematic aspects of communication, they may also develop in the course of the interaction. This emphasises the emergent and negotiable features of the interaction.

In emphasising the negotiable aspects of the consultation, however, we do not pretend that the strategies are enacted in an open arena. There are three limits on the possibilities for action. First, there is the limitation on the interaction imposed by the organisation of medical care in this country. The patient usually sees just one doctor for primary medical care and has limited ability to change doctors. Furthermore, the patient is somewhat limited in his possibilities for action in that he perceives his knowledge, and the information available to him, to be of a different order from that of the professional. We deal with these problems more fully in the final chapters.

A second limit is in the actors' perceptions of what is possible. Thus patients may perceive that they are constrained by the amount of time available for the consultation, or they may feel constrained because the interaction takes place on the doctor's territory.

The third limitation to the strategic interaction concerns areas of implicit agreement in interaction. Order in the consultation is maintained by complicity, by agreements on the way certain aspects of the encounter are to be managed: such things as the use of jokes, the modes of address each use, the emotional flatness of the consultation and the use of reassurance and empathy. Such aspects might, in lay terms, be summed up as 'good manners'.

What it is important to realise with these limitations to negotiation is *not* that the above are not all negotiable – for example, the patient can insist that the doctor devotes more time to the problem – but that they are *less* negotiable than other aspects of the consultation.

Presenting a problem to the doctor

In discussing the patient's prognosis in the consultation, a report from a working party of the Royal College of General Practitioners (1972) advises the doctor to ask himself certain questions:

> What must I tell this patient? How much of what I learned about him should he know? What words shall I use to convey this information? How much of what I propose to tell him will he understand? How will he react? How much of my advice will he take? What degree of pressure am I entitled to apply? (p. 17).

If we change the second from last of these questions to read, 'How much notice will he take of what I say?' then these could be exactly the questions that the patient poses to himself when seeing the doctor. For the patient considers, both prior to and during the consultation, *what to say* to the doctor. Under this heading we deal with the patient's interpretation and selection of facts and the ways in which he attempts to put these across to the doctor with the maximum effect.

In perceiving his symptoms, the patient attempts to *interpret* them, and in explaining these symptoms both to himself and to the doctor, he is defining, categorising and causally linking them to other factors which he feels may be related. Thus the disorder may be presented in conjunction with another physical condition that the patient believes to be relevant. One woman explained her problem to the doctor in this way: 'I've had a lot of headaches lately – I wondered if it could be anything to do with my blood pressure?' The symptoms may be described in terms of a social context which the patient sees as significant, e.g. the woman patient who told the doctor she believed her anxiety and 'nerves' stemmed from her worries about a delinquent daughter. This interpreting is partly an attempt at self-diagnosis and partly an attempt to 'put the doctor on the right lines'. What is significant to the patient may not be so for the doctor, who may dismiss the patient's perceptions and interpretations as having little relevance and may probe for other factors that the patient has not mentioned. Strauss *et al.* (1964) give an example of this situation among patients in a psychiatric hospital who cannot understand the approach of their doctors. One patient was troubled:

> . . . by what the doctor considered important and the kinds of judgement the doctor made. What he himself considered important and talked about at length, the doctor usually dismissed as unimportant. What he thought trivial the doctor might seize upon (p. 268).

As well, therefore, as having to define or recognise a problem and putting this into words, the patient is also involved in 'figuring out' the doctor. Both parties are 'sizing each other up'. The patient may not agree with the doctor's interpretation of his symptoms, especially when this does not accord with his own preconceived ideas and the doctor has not stated his interpretation in terms sufficiently convincing to persuade the patient to accept it.

References

Maddox, E.J. (1973), 'The Diagnostic Process: a sociological approach to some factors affecting outcomes with special reference to variation', Aberdeen University: Master's thesis.

Marinker, M. (1970), 'Truce', in M. Balint *et al.* (1970) *Treatment or Diagnosis: A Study of Repeat Prescriptions in General Practice,* London: Tavistock Publications, ch. 7.

Mauksch, H.O. (1972), 'Ideology, interaction and patient care in hospitals'; paper presented at the Third International Conference on Social Science and Medicine, Elsinore, Denmark.

Roth, J.A. (1963), *Timetables: Structuring the Passage of Time in Hospital Treatment and other Careers*, Indianapolis: Bobbs-Merrill.

Royal College of General Practitioners Working Party (1972), *The Future General Practitioner*, London: Royal College of General Practitioners.

Scheff, T.J. (1968) 'Negotiating reality: notes on power in the assessment of responsibility', *Social Problems*, 16, 1, pp. 3–17.

Strauss, A., Schatzman, L., Bucher, R., Ehrlich, D. and Sabshin, M. (1964), *Psychiatric Ideologies and Institutions*, London: Collier-Macmillan.

Strong, P.M. and Davis, A.G. (1972), 'Problems and strategies in a paediatric clinic'; paper presented at the Third International Conference on Social Science and Medicine, Elsinore, Denmark.

27 Managing courtesy stigma

The case of Alzheimer's disease*

Hazel MacRae

Introduction

Most studies of stigma have focused on the experiences of persons who possess a discrediting attribute or condition, with attention usually given to strategies they employ in an effort to protect their precarious identities. What Goffman has termed 'courtesy stigma' has received much less research attention. Goffman argues that there is a 'tendency for stigma to spread from the stigmatized individual to his [sic] close connections . . .' (1963: 30). When an individual 'is related through the social structure to a stigmatized individual', the wider society may then 'treat both individuals in some respects as one' (Goffman 1963: 30). Citing examples such as 'the loyal spouse of the mental patient' and 'the daughter of the ex-con', Goffman argues that these individuals 'are obliged to share some of the discredit of the stigmatized person to whom they are related' (1963: 30). Family members of persons who have a stigmatising illness, then, may experience stigmatisation 'because of their affiliation with the stigmatised individual rather than through any characteristic of their own' (Gray 1993: 104). This paper investigates whether family members of persons diagnosed with Alzheimer's disease experience stigma, examines strategies of stigma management, and explains why some persons are able to avoid stigmatisation while others are not. [. . .]

Courtesy stigma and Alzheimer's disease

There are some studies of Alzheimer's disease and other types of dementia where researchers have noted that relatives and caregivers reported that they often felt embarrassed by the behaviours of their ill family member (Greene *et al.* 1982, Argyle *et al.* 1985, Fontana and Smith 1989). Moreover, while there are not many studies which focus directly on the topic of Alzheimer's disease and stigma, there are a few exceptions (Schifflet and Blieszner 1988, Blum 1991). Of these studies, Blum's deserves mention since her research focused directly on courtesy stigma among Alzheimer family caregivers.

*This is an abridged version of an article that was first published in *Sociology of Health & Illness*, vol. 21, no. 1, pp. 54–70, 1999.

According to Blum's findings, stigma management by Alzheimer caregivers moves through two phases. In the first phase, the caregiver colludes with the ill family member as they cooperate in the management of information and problematic situations. 'The caregiver becomes a partner in passing, helping to preserve both the public face of the family member and of the family (or "couple") as a collective unit' (1991: 267). Passing involves concealment of damaging information or the management of undisclosed discrediting inform-ation (Goffman 1963: 42). The caregiver and the person with Alzheimer's disease also engage in what Goffman has termed 'covering'. Covering practices are employed where the stigma becomes visible or is known about but effort is made to keep it from 'looming large' (Goffman 1963: 102). As Blum explains, 'as the stigma becomes visible in interaction, the caregiver makes efforts to minimise its salience. Thus covering involves situation management, such that the visibility of the trouble and the embarrassment it may cause are kept to a minimum' (1991: 270). When the competence of the person with Alzheimers diminishes and he/she 'can no longer play the collusive game', the second phase begins. Information control is no longer the main concern: the primary concern now is to prevent or manage the problematic situations that arise as a result of the ill family member's inappropriate behaviour. The caregiver now 'realigns and sides against the family member in order to maintain social order as well as preserve his or her own face' (1991: 281–2). [. . .]

This paper's contribution to the literature is twofold. First, it expands the research focus beyond primary caregivers to include other family members. Previous research has shown that caring for someone who has Alzheimer's disease is stressful but little is known about how family members who are not caregivers are affected by this disease. Blum's study illustrates that Alzheimer caregivers experience courtesy stigma; this study illustrates that other family members may be affected by courtesy stigma as well. Second, the findings of this study are important because they show that not all family members perceive themselves to be stigmatised, and the paper outlines some of the factors that influence the experience of stigma.

Methods

The sample for this study consisted of 47 family members of persons diag-nosed with probable Alzheimer's disease. Thirty-one were primary caregivers; fourteen of these were spousal caregivers and seventeen adult-child caregivers. The remaining 16 respondents were all children of persons with Alzheimer's disease; 11 were children of the spousal caregivers, four were children of spousal caregivers who were not part of the study; the remaining respondent was the sibling of an adult-child caregiver. The majority of the participants were located through the assistance of physicians and nurses at a medical centre in the province of Nova Scotia where patients with Alzheimer's disease are diagnosed and assessed at regular intervals. Two respondents volunteered after seeing a notice about the study that had been placed in a newsletter of the Alzheimer Society of Nova Scotia. Two others became part of the sample when their names were given to the researcher by a respondent who had been interviewed earlier.

The data were gathered in semi-structured, in-depth, tape-recorded interviews. The majority of the respondents were interviewed in their homes; however, two chose to have the interview conducted in a coffee shop. While all of the primary caregivers were interviewed individually, of the other family members interviewed, two pairs of sisters were interviewed together. Basically, three questions were used to investigate the experience of stigma and strategies of stigma management. Respondents were asked if they had ever tried to cover up or disguise the memory loss or other disabilities of the family member who had Alzheimers. If they had, they were asked about the kinds of strategies they had employed. They were asked whether they had ever been embarrassed or felt ashamed because of their ill family member's behaviour. And, they were asked whether they had ever avoided certain situations or going places with their spouse or parent where they thought they might be embarrassed. The first question was designed to elicit information concerning efforts to normalise or to use information management as a way of hopefully preventing a stigmatising situation. The purpose of the last two questions was to establish whether respondents had experienced stigma and/or fearing it, tried to avoid potentially discrediting situations.

It is important to emphasise that this is a qualitative study and although some numerical data are reported, numbers should be interpreted with caution since the sample is small and not random. Also, it is difficult in many instances to make generalisations because there was considerable variation among the persons diagnosed with Alzheimer's disease in terms of the extent to which the disease had progressed, and the related degree of disability and change in behaviour. In the early period, symptoms are often not all that visible to others. In fact, often it is only an intimate other who will recognise any sign of disease at all. On the other hand, in the later stages symptoms can be quite severe and behavioural changes dramatic. Also, at any point along its course, there can be marked variation in symptomatology among persons who have this disease (see Gubrium 1986). Therefore, some persons with Alzheimer's disease are less difficult to deal with than others and discrediting information is more easily concealed. This is a factor to be considered in trying to make sense of variation in the data.

Findings

Consistent with previous research, the findings of this study reveal that when one member of a family has a stigmatised illness other members are at risk of acquiring courtesy stigma. And, aware of their potential fate, they use various strategies of stigma management. Some are seemingly able to escape stigma altogether, while others work at managing problematic situations once they have occurred. Many respondents recounted embarrassing incidents during which they experienced shame. What is most noteworthy, however, is the finding that a substantial number of others did not appear to have experienced stigma and/or claimed not to have ever been embarrassed or ashamed. In addition very few respondents (30 per cent of spousal caregivers, 29 per cent of child caregivers, 25 per cent of the noncaregiving children) said that they avoided going places or situations where they feared they might be embarrassed. [. . .]

Escaping stigmatisation and strategies of stigma management

Since definitions of the situation are negotiated rather than given, affiliation with a stigmatised individual does not automatically result in courtesy stigma. The data analysis in this section will show that family members of persons with Alzheimer's disease can avoid stigma if they are able to manipulate or control the definition of the situation so that others' reactions will not be negative. Some families use information control so that the discreditable condition is rendered invisible, concealability being a crucial factor. Others control the reactions of others either by medicalising the problem or using a technique of neutralisation. The relevant factor here is family members' ability to either challenge or ignore the other's definition of the situation and rely on their own interpretation of the meaning of the potentially stigmatising condition. In the final situation, the relevant factor is the availability of 'supportive others' who, although aware of the discreditable condition, are sympathetic and nonjudgemental.

Covering up the discreditable condition

Concealability is a 'critically important dimension of stigma' (Jones *et al.* 1984: 29) that refers to the visibility of the attribute or condition and thus whether or not it is easily detected. In this study, concealability is one of the most important factors influencing stigma avoidance and management. And, whether concealment is used as a means to manage stigma is related to the nature of the relationship between the person with Alzheimer's disease and the potentially stigmatised family member (i.e. whether the family member is a spouse or child and/or a primary caregiver) and the visibility of symptoms.

Similar to Blum's (1991) findings, there is evidence of a collusive alignment between the caregiver and the person with Alzheimer's disease, and there are numerous examples which indicate that both passing and covering practices were used to influence favourably others' definitions of the situation so as to accomplish stigma management. Eleven of the 14 spousal caregivers claimed that they had tried to disguise their spouse's memory loss or other disabilities. And, among their responses there is evidence that caregiving spouses colluded with their husbands or wives in the management of potentially discrediting situations. As an example of the practice of passing, the following respondent explains how she co-operated with her husband to conceal his forgetfulness:

> Yes, someone would come and say 'hello', they'd say, 'how are you doing Fred?' He would say, 'fine'. He'd look at me and I'd say, 'I can't remember your name'; then they'd say who they were.

[. . .]

Concealability is related to another factor that influences experience of stigma-variation in symptomatology. In their study of relatives of former mental patients, Freeman and Simmons (1975) report that stigma was associated with severity of symptoms or the degree of bizarre behaviour on the part of the patient. The more bizarre the behaviour, the more difficult it is to conceal. As Schneider and Conrad (1980) illustrate in their study of epilepsy, the stigma potential of some conditions is greater than others because some conditions are more visible (see also Crocker *et al.* 1993). The stigma potential of Alzheimer's disease generally increases as the disease advances and symptoms become more severe and more difficult to conceal. However, when symptoms are not severe and thus less visible, it is possible to manage the stigma and even avoid it.

Some of the respondents in this study were able to escape stigmatisation because symptoms were fewer and less severe (e.g. some memory loss versus going outdoors without clothes on) and the ill family member's behaviour was not disruptive. That severity of symptoms and visibility influence stigma is evident in the typical qualified response of a son who said he had never tried to cover up his mother's illness: 'no, her social skills are still intact'. [. . .]

Medicalisation of deviance: misbehaviour as disease

It is generally held that the afflicted person's role in producing the potentially stigmatising condition is an important factor in the stigmatising process (Jones *et al.* 1984, Ainlay *et al.* 1986, Rodin *et al.* 1989). Individuals who are judged to be not responsible for their condition are less likely to be stigmatised. Even though there is not complete agreement within the medical community concerning the nature of Alzheimer's disease as a disease, a biomedical paradigm is generally used as a framework for explaining the nature of the disorder (see, Gubrium 1986, Lyman 1993). When individuals are officially diagnosed, the condition is presented as an organic disease 'said to be "caused" by the degeneration of the cells of the brain' (Gubrium 1986: 18). The biomedical model is also ubiquitous within what Gubrium calls the 'public culture' or 'growing body of public understandings about the disease' (1986: 111).

If Alzheimers is viewed as an organically-based disease, then, inappropriate or unusual behaviour, behaviour that would otherwise be considered deviant, can be interpreted as merely a symptom of disease. Deviant behaviour is medicalised and the individual is absolved of responsibility for his or her actions. Within the Alzheimer disease literature, in particular within the caregiver handbooks (see, for example, Mace and Rabins 1981), caregivers are told they must always remember that persons with this disease are not responsible for their actions. They are instructed to remember that whatever the afflicted individual does that is 'out of character' is a result of the disease; behavioural outbursts are a manifestation of the disease, 'not the real person' (Gubrium 1986: 93).

Almost all the persons interviewed in this study had read some literature on Alzheimer's disease and it was obvious that most had been exposed to its 'public culture'. For example, almost everyone used the stage theory (i.e. supposedly there are 'typical' stages of decline) to explain the extent to which the disease had progressed in their loved one. And, some of the respondents employed a medicalisation of deviance strategy to avoid and/or manage stigma. For example, a caregiving daughter said that she had never tried to cover up her mother's disabilities, nor had she ever been ashamed, because her mother had an *illness*:

> No never, never. There's nothing to be ashamed of and I think if people are going to cope with it, they have to know [that she has Alzheimers] and people are going to have to understand my mother. They have to know definitely just what's wrong.

[. . .]

Condemning the condemners

A number of respondents, all adult-children, refused to become victims of stigmatisation by using a technique of neutralisation. Basically, according to their definition of the situation, if others were uncomfortable in the presence of the person with Alzheimer's disease, that was *their* problem. Moreover, these family members typically took the position that people who react negatively 'don't count' anyway. For example, when asked if she had ever tried to conceal her father's memory loss or other disabilities, a daughter who was caring for her father, said:

> No, people have to accept him the way he is . . . , and if they don't know him well enough to realize that there is something wrong then they don't count.

Similarly, another caregiving daughter, when asked whether she had ever experienced embarrassment or shame because of her mother's behaviour, stated:

> Yes, and well people say the strangest things to you. One of the women . . . , who had met mum once or twice, just came right out and said, 'your mother should be in a nursing home.' And, people like that, you just write them off as acquaintances altogether.

[. . .]

Availability of supportive others and situational variability

According to Jones *et al.* (1984), one variable that influences stigma is the degree of social distance between the person with the discrediting condition and the audience making the judgement about his or her behaviour. Social distance refers to the degree of familiarity between the participants in an interaction and is related to the degree of interpersonal involvement between them. People at a close relational distance are less likely to stigmatise. According to the definition of relational distance, an individual's family and kin would presumably be at the closest relational distance, followed by friends, neighbours and acquaintances (Jones *et al.* 1984). Some respondents in this study explained that they had not ever found themselves in a potentially embarrassing situation, usually because most of the contact they had with the ill family took place inside the family setting (e.g. 'she hasn't been out of the house for three years'). Supportive family members, then, can 'serve as a protective circle' (Goffman 1963: 97) so that within the confines of the home there is less reason to be concerned about embarrassment and little need to engage in stigma management.

Other family members were able to escape stigmatisation because of the availability of nonfamilial supportive others who were 'in the know' but granted 'consideration' (Birenbaum 1970). 'Consideration' is received when others show a 'polite recognition and acceptance of the plight' of a family with a person who has Alzheimer's disease. Consideration 'means that the situation will never be spoken about unless brought up' (Birenbaum 1970: 199) by the family members themselves. Stigma can be managed if encounters are limited to supportive friends and neighbours; relations with neighbours and friends who are not considerate can be avoided and/or terminated (Birenbaum 1970). [. . .]

Discussion

The findings of this study confirm earlier work which has shown that familial caregivers to persons with Alzheimer's disease experience courtesy stigma. In addition, the data show that it is not only caregivers who experience courtesy stigma and employ strategies of stigma management but other family members as well. Important is the finding that a good number of the family members claimed not to have experienced stigma and did not appear to be concerned about trying to avoid it. The findings illustrate the complexity of the stigma issue and the intricacies involved in the special case of stigma and Alzheimer's disease.

The analysis indicates that further empirical and conceptual work on the concept of courtesy stigma and the factors that influence its occurrence is needed. Goffman (1963) outlined in detail the processes by which a stigma is acquired but says much less about how courtesy stigma develops. As he described it, courtesy stigma is simply *acquired* by virtue of the individual's relationship to the person who possesses a stigma. But, as the findings of this study illustrate, some individuals who are closely related to a stigmatised person do not perceive themselves to be stigmatised, even in potentially stigmatising situations. Further research investigating the conditions under which some individuals succumb to courtesy stigma while others seemingly 'fight back' would make an important contribution to current knowledge about stigma.

Contemplating why some persons are able to escape stigma while others are not, Vaz speculates that 'the ability to successfully reject the censure of others (however systematic it may be) is surely related to the availability of strategic resources and the ability to organize them successfully' (1976: 80). The findings of this study show that an individual's capacity as an actor to reject the other's definition of the situation and interpret a potentially stigmatising condition as a legitimate medical illness is one strategic resource. However, further research is needed that investigates the part individuals play in the definition of the meaning of illness and what distinguishes those who are able to challenge others' definitions of the situation from those who are not. Moreover, it would be useful to know something about the general public's understanding of Alzheimer's disease. Presumably the more knowledgeable others are, the greater the likelihood that they will accept the 'beyond-[his or her]-control medical interpretation' (Schneider and Conrad, 1980: 41) of a potentially discrediting event.

As these study findings have shown, it is possible to avoid the courtesy stigma of Alzheimer's disease if symptoms of the disease are concealed from others. Collusion and cover up are, however, stressful and may involve avoidance of face-to-face contact with others which entails a further cost of decreasing social contact for the person who has the disease and possibly increased isolation for an already increasingly housebound familial caregiver. In addition, while concealment may be a successful stigma avoidance strategy, it works for only as long as the person with Alzheimer's disease is willing and able to cooperate in covering up the potentially discreditable condition. Thus, 'covering up' is only a short-term option, for as the disease eventually progresses its visibility inevitably increases and a new strategy must be devised if family members are to avoid becoming the victims of courtesy stigma.

References

Ainlay, S., Becker, G. and Coleman, L. (eds) (1986) *The Dilemma of Difference*. New York: Plenum Press.

Argyle, N., Jestice, S. and Brook, C. (1985) Psychogeriatric patients: their supporters' problems, *Age and Ageing*, 14, 355–60

Birenbaum, A. (1970) On managing a courtesy stigma, *Journal of Health and Social Behaviour*, 11, 196–206.

Blum, N.S. (1991) The management of stigma by Alzheimer family caregivers, *Journal of Contemporary Ethnography*, 20, 263–84.

Crocker, J., Cornwell, B. and Major, B. (1993) The stigma of overweight: affective consequences of attributional ambiguity, *Journal of Personality and Social Psychology*, 64, 6–70.

Fontana, A. and Smith, R.W. (1989) Alzheimer disease victims: the 'Unbecoming' of self and the normalization of competence, *Sociological Perspective*, 32, 47–64.

Freeman, H. and Simmons, O. (1975) Feelings of stigma among relatives of former mental patients. In Scarpitti, F. and McFarlane, P. (eds) *Deviance: Action, Reaction, Interaction*. Reading, Massachusetts: Addison-Wesley.

Goffman, E. (1963) *Stigma*. Englewood Cliffs, New Jersey: Prentice Hall.

Gray, D. (1993) Perceptions of stigma: the parents of autistic children, *Sociology of Health and Illness*, 15, 102–20.

Greene, J.G., Smith, R., Gardiner, M. and Timbury, G.C. (1982) Measuring behaviourial disturbance of elderly demented patients in the community and its effects on relatives: a factor analytic study, *Age and Ageing*, 11, 121–6.

Gubrium, J. (1986) *Oldtimers and Alzheimers: the Descriptive Organization of Senility*. Greenwich, Connecticut: Jai Press.

Jones, E., Farina, A., Hastorf, A., Markus, H., Miller, D. and Scott, R. (1984) *Social Stigma*. New York: W. H. Freeman and Company.

Lyman, K. (1993) *Day In, Day Out with Alzheimer's: Stress in Caregiving Relationships*. Philadelphia: Temple University Press.

Mace, N.L. and Rabins, P.V. (1981) *The 36-Hour Day*. Baltimore: Johns Hopkins University Press.

Rodin, M., Price, J., Sanchez, F. and McElligot, S. (1989) Derogation, exclusion, and unfair treatment of persons with social flaws: controllability of stigma and the attribution of prejudice, *Personality and Social Psychology Bulletin*, 15, 439–51.

Schneider, J.W. and Conrad, P. (1980) In the closet with illness: epilepsy, stigma potential and information control, *Social Problems*, 28, 32–44.

Schifflet, P. and Blieszner, R. (1988) Stigma and Alzheimer's disease: behaviourial consequences for support groups, *The Journal of Applied Gerontology*, 7, 147–60.

Vaz, E. (1976) *Aspects of Deviance*. Scarborough, Ontario: Prentice Hall.

28 Researching women's health work*

Hilary Graham

Introducing the study: the social and material contexts of health-related behaviour

The study of mothers on income support is drawn from a larger survey of smoking patterns among lone and cohabiting mothers caring for babies of six months old (Graham 1993). The original survey was drawn from the records of two maternity hospitals and included White and African-Caribbean mothers in households where the head of household was either unemployed/economically inactive or was employed in a manual occupation.[1] The majority (96 per cent) of the mothers identified themselves as White. Among the mothers who took part in the study, 242 were dependent, in whole or in part, on income support.[2] It is this group of mothers whose lives and lifestyles are the focus of this and the subsequent section.

The majority of the mothers on income support were under the age of twenty-five and were caring for children outside a cohabiting relationship with a male or female partner (Figures 1 and 2). Reflecting the younger age of their children, the proportion of single (never married) women is higher, and the proportion of separated and divorced women is lower, than in the general population of mothers on income support (Department of Social Security 1994).

Mothers' lives were structured around the daily routines of caring for young children. Only three mothers (1 per cent) reported that they were not with and caring for their baby on a full-time basis. A substantial minority (43 per cent) were caring for other pre-school children as well and, again, almost all were doing so on a full-time basis. Paid employment provided a break from childcare for less than one in ten (7 per cent) of the mothers. Mothers' domestic responsibilities extended beyond the routine provision of childcare to include the care of partners and children with acute and chronic illness or who experienced some form of impairment. Over a third (37 per cent) of the babies were reported to have a persistent cough and nearly half (47 per cent) had a persistent cold.

*This is an extract from the chapter 'Researching women's health work: a study of the lifestyles of mothers on income support' first published in Bywaters, P. and McLeod, E. (eds) (1996) *Working for Equality in Health*, Routledge, pp. 161–78.

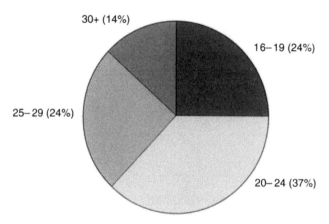

Figure 1 Age of mothers (*n*=242).

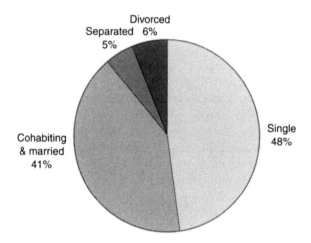

Figure 2 Cohabitation status of mothers (*n*=242).

Indicators regarded as a sensitive measure of the living standards of white women, like housing tenure, suggest that the majority of the mothers in the study were working for health without access to the material resources that most families take for granted. Nationally, 35 per cent of lone parent families and 76 per cent of two parent families are living in owner-occupied housing (Office of Population Censuses and Surveys 1991). Among the mothers in the study, only one in five (22 per cent) were in owner-occupied housing, with single women living with their parents making up a large proportion of this group. It should be noted that tenure provides a static measure of what was often an insecure and unstable housing situation, as the following accounts illustrate:

He (partner) had an accident at work and broke his wrist. He has had metal pins inserted. It happened about Christmas and he is still out of work. He shared his house with his sister and her husband, so when I became pregnant, there wasn't enough room and we had to find somewhere else to live. We thought we might have to go into bed and breakfast. We got this house about a week before she (daughter) was born. We were quite lucky really.

My husband's been sick and out of work for 18 months. He managed to get a job here but no accommodation. We're renting but it's expensive and the tenancy finishes in December and we'll be homeless if we can't find anywhere else. We've no money for our own home and we'll be back in bed and breakfast again.

(cohabiting mothers)

Other measures of environmental conditions suggest that mothers were caring for children in homes and neighbourhoods in which health hazards were a routine feature (Figure 3). Half of the mothers (51 per cent) reported that dangerous roads were a problem and the same proportion identified a lack of play space for children in the neighbourhood. Over half of the mothers also reported dogs as neighbourhood problems, with a third reporting litter and vandalism as problems. While their homes and neighbourhoods lacked the space in which their children could play, and play safely, few mothers had private transport to enable them to use facilities further away. Less than one in three mothers (30 per cent) lived in a household with a car or van. A significantly smaller proportion had access to this household resource. Only one in six (15 per cent) of the sample had access to a car/van during week days. While not a substitute for private transport, household ownership of a

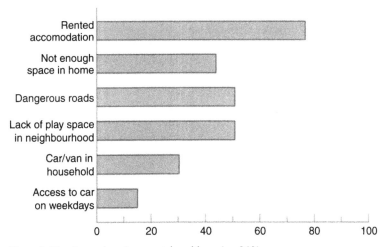

Figure 3 Housing and environmental problems (*n*=242).

telephone can offset the effects of transport deprivation, providing mothers with a way of accessing health care routinely and in emergencies. However, the majority of the mothers (51 per cent) lived in accommodation without a telephone.

More subjective measures of living standards again suggest that the mothers were working for health in circumstances that denied them access to the material resources they needed. One of the questions asked mothers to assess how well their households were coping financially: to indicate whether their household was able to pay for all the things it needed, most of the things it needed, some of the things or hardly any of the things. Only one in five mothers (21 per cent) reported that their family was able to pay for all the necessities. The majority (57 per cent) noted that they were able to afford some or hardly any of the things they needed. In the struggle to make ends meet, items of personal expenditure, like clothes, were sacrificed to protect the living standards of their families. Thus, while the majority reported that they usually had enough money for food for their family (87 per cent) and for clothes for their children (70 per cent), only a minority of mothers (37 per cent) usually had enough money to pay for clothes for themselves.

> Bills are a problem. The problem is really when the money situation gets you really depressed, you might go out and buy something like some nice beefburgers and that makes it worse. We've got rent arrears of over £1,000 now. Every week the amount goes up.
>
> We've so many debts we don't know what to do.
>
> Fear of eviction is our biggest problem. It's still on-going. We have to go to court. If we can guarantee to pay they probably won't evict us. And the poll tax is a big problem. I received a letter saying they would take me to court as I hadn't paid it. I missed two payments.
>
> (cohabiting mothers)

The circumstances in which mothers were working for health were not only constrained by material shortages and insecurities. Mothers were also often labouring for health with limited health resources of their own. When asked to assess their health as excellent, good, fair or poor, only one in eight (12 per cent) rated it as excellent; four in ten (39 per cent) assessed their health as fair or poor. The national *Health and Lifestyle Survey* provides comparative data on women aged 18 to 49 in households with high weekly incomes. In this group, 25 per cent rated their health as excellent and 16 per cent assessed it as fair to poor (Cox 1987).

Poor self-assessed health reflected the experience of a range of chronic health problems across the two weeks prior to the interview, like being constantly tired and having backache and headaches (Figure 4). It was also linked to the experience of long-term illness and physical impairment. One in four (26 per cent) reported long-standing illness or physical impairment, with

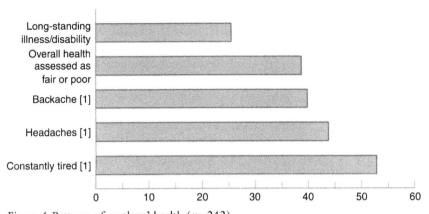

Figure 4 Patterns of mothers' health (*n*=242).
Note [1] within the two weeks prior to interview.

asthma, impaired hearing and impaired movement (including arthritis and back and hip problems) figuring prominently in the mothers' replies.

The findings summarized in this section suggest that caring in the face of limited material resources and limited health resources provided the context within which health-related behaviours were sustained.

Working for health through health-damaging behaviours?

The routines of caring for children rest on behaviours which have become a focus of surveillance and intervention by health professionals, including infant feeding and cigarette smoking. The survey confirmed the socio-economic patterning of these targeted behaviours. Reflecting the youthful age profile of the mothers, initial rates of breast feeding were slightly below national prevalence rates for mothers in social class V and lone mothers (see Figure 5). Among mothers who initially breast fed, patterns of breast feeding at one month are in line with national rates among mothers in the poorest material circumstances (see Figure 5).

Smoking patterns are summarized in Table 1. The majority (61 per cent) of the mothers reported that they smoked one or more cigarettes a day, with smokers clustered amongst those with relatively high rates of cigarette consumption. Seventeen per cent of the smokers reported that they smoked

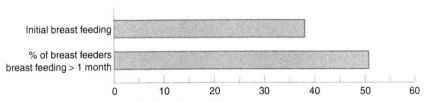

Figure 5 Patterns of breast feeding (*n*=242).

Table 1 Patterns of cigarette smoking (*n*=242).

	%	(*n*)
Current smokers		
Less than 10 a day	17	(23)
10–19 a day	43	(64)
20+ a day	41	(61)
Total current smokers	61	
Ex-regular smokers	13	(32)
Never or only occasionally smoked a cigarette	26	(62)
		(242)

less than ten cigarettes a day, while more than 40 per cent smoked twenty plus cigarettes a day. In the general population of female smokers aged 16 to 34, the proportion of light smokers is significantly higher (26 per cent) and the proportion smoking more than twenty cigarettes a day is significantly lower (28 per cent) (Office of Population Censuses and Surveys 1994).

High rates of prevalence and consumption were matched by low rates of never-smoking. Only one in four (26 per cent) of the mothers had never smoked: in the general population of women aged 16 to 34, the proportion is 54 per cent (Office of Population Censuses and Surveys 1994).

These smoking habits were sustained in the face of knowledge of the health risks of smoking. When asked if they thought that smoking was bad for people's health, 84 per cent of the mothers gave an unqualified yes. When those who qualified their answer is some way are included, the proportion rises to over 90 per cent. A lower proportion agreed that parental smoking was bad for the health of children. None the less, over 70 per cent gave an unqualified yes to the question; a proportion that rose to over 80 per cent when those who qualified their answer are included.

In contrast to their smoking behaviour, the drinking habits of mothers on income support were well within the limits prescribed by Government. Mothers noted how they cut down or gave up drinking in pregnancy and that, while they typically resumed their pre-pregnancy levels of drinking after birth, levels of consumption were generally low (Figure 6). The majority (62 per cent) of the mothers reported that they drank less than once a week. Only a small minority (3 per cent) reported drinking more than twice a week. These patterns stand in sharp contrast to those recorded by men in low-income households. National surveys suggest that nearly nine in ten (86 per cent) of men aged 18 to 39 in low-income households have at least one drink a week. Nearly half report drinking moderately or heavily (Cox 1987).

Mothers' accounts of their smoking habits and drinking habits suggest that they formed part of a broader lifestyle fashioned out of the needs and constraints of caring for children on income support. While smoking cigarettes formed an integral part of this lifestyle, drinking alcohol was rarely

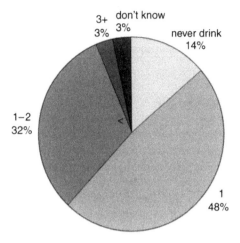

Figure 6 Patterns of alcohol consumption (times per week) (*n*=242).

part of the daily routine through which they tried to keep themselves and their families going. The difference in the meanings and contexts of these two patterns of behaviour is illustrated in the answers mothers gave to questions about when they were likely to smoke and to have an alcoholic drink.

When smokers were asked to identify any times and situations when they were very likely to smoke, the most common response was to describe structured and anticipated breaks from caring, when, if even for a few minutes, mothers could rest and refuel. For example, nearly half (47 per cent) of the smokers described routine breaks as times in which they were very likely to smoke; a similar proportion (44 per cent) also identified situations when they could relax. Nearly three in four (73 per cent) said they were very likely to smoke if they got a bit of time to themselves during the day. Their accounts suggest that, along with a cup of tea or coffee, smoking a cigarette gave access to personal space and adult time. These moments of relaxation could also mark out a social life beyond childcare, with cigarettes given and shared with partners, family and friends.

> *Times or situations mothers identified as ones in which they were very likely to want to smoke*
>
> In the evening, sometimes I can sit down. I'm always on the go but I grab one when I sit down.
>
> In the afternoon when she has gone to bed and I can sit down for a few minutes.
>
> When I have a cup of tea and when my mum comes over. When I'm drinking, I'm more inclined to smoke. When my husband smokes.
>
> (cohabiting mothers)

When I get five minutes from the kids.

At night, when the kids are in bed, that's when I enjoy one. First thing in the morning, but mainly at night.

(lone mothers)

Cigarette smoking was not only a habit structured by the demands and routines of caring. It was a habit deeply woven into the *process* of caring, providing a way of managing and defusing stress. Childcare situations which mothers found stressful were the second most common context mothers described when asked the open-ended question about particular times and situations in which they were very likely to smoke. Answers to a follow-up question about smoking in the context of feeling on edge underlined the stress-management function of smoking. Nine in ten mothers (87 per cent) stated that they would be very likely to smoke if they were feeling on edge and needed to calm their nerves.

> *Times or situations mothers identified as ones in which they were very likely to smoke*
>
> I have noticed when something gets on top of me, I light a fag up and relax.
>
> When the baby is screaming and won't shut up.
>
> When my eldest son won't do as he's told and he answers me back.
>
> When I'm making the tea. The two older ones come home from school, the baby's hungry and all four of them are hungry. They are all fighting and screaming and the dinner's cooking in the kitchen. I'm ready to blow up so I light a cigarette. It calms me down when I'm under so much stress.

(cohabiting mothers)

Smoking as a stress reduction strategy also figured prominently in the accounts that mothers gave for increases in consumption. For example, two mothers explained why they smoked more in pregnancy in the following way:

> I more or less chain-smoked (in pregnancy). It was the other kids who caused the stress. I had three under 4 years and I was pregnant. It was just the pressures from the children. The worry about everything got me down. The kids, the house, the shopping. The worry about how I was going to cope with the new baby, having him so close to the others.

(cohabiting mother)

> Coping with the babies. I wasn't able to cope with two of them on my own, with my husband away (in prison).

(lone mother)

As mothers' accounts suggest, cigarette smoking was a coping strategy to which mothers had direct and immediate access. It was experienced as a habit that helped mothers fulfil their domestic responsibilities, both on a routine basis and through the times of stress that punctuate the lives of women caring for young children. Its distinctive place in mothers' lives is underlined when accounts of smoking and drinking habits are compared. Very few mothers identified either the ordinary routines of childcare or coping with situations where their children were getting 'out of hand' as ones in which they would be very likely to drink. In contrast to the 73 per cent of smokers who said they would be very likely to have a cigarette if they got a bit of time to themselves during the day, only 1 per cent of the mothers who drank alcohol identified having time to themselves as a situation in which they were very likely to drink. A similarly small proportion (1 per cent) of the drinkers stated that they would be very likely to drink at times when their children were getting 'out of hand' and they were having difficulty coping. More drinkers (5 per cent) reported that they would be very likely to drink if they were feeling on edge and needed to calm their nerves. However, the proportion is still significantly below the 87 per cent of smokers who said that they would be very likely to smoke in this situation. Instead of being meshed into the routines and stresses of caring, having a drink appeared to be associated with times and locations where mothers were away from domestic responsibilities and from the domestic contexts in which they worked to meet them:

> I go out occasionally with some friends up the street. It sounds awful going out but a group of us go to the pub about once in a couple of weeks. The men can go any time, any night, any Sunday.

> When I was pregnant, I thought it was bad for the baby. I can have a drink now if I fancy it but I don't go out much. I don't drink in the house.

> Before I had the baby, I was out every night of the week. Now I only go out once a week. I feel as if I want to drink to make my night. It makes me feel it's an evening off.

> (cohabiting mothers)

Conclusions

For over a century, individual behaviour has been identified as a major cause of ill health and premature death in Britain. Maternal behaviour has figured particularly centrally in debates about the nation's health, with the unhealthy habits of mothers identified as the major cause of disease and death in childhood in the early decades of the century (Lewis 1980; Smith and Nicholson 1992).

As in the past, a lifestyle emphasis is strongly in evidence in today's health policies, with interventions framed in ways which separate individual behaviour from its social and material context. This chapter, however, has turned the spotlight on these contexts, using sociological research to explore the connections between living conditions and lifestyles. It has focused on a study of mothers on income support who were working for health at home.

The study suggests that the mothers' lives were structured by their 'health work' and are framed by their material circumstances. Health-related behaviours were woven into lives characterized by heavy caring responsibilities, poor health and limited access to material resources. Some behaviours, like alcohol consumption, occupied a marginal place in the routines that sustained mothers through each day. It was identified as a habit which, while health-damaging, was not essential to their survival. Cigarette smoking, in contrast, was seen as a deeply contradictory habit, which both undermined and promoted the welfare of their family. On the one hand, mothers recognized the health costs of smoking, for themselves and their children. On the other, they were aware of its pivotal place in the routines which kept them going, hour by hour and day by day. Cigarette smoking was experienced as a child-protective strategy, a resource which helped mothers cope with the demands of caring, both on a routine basis and through the periods of stress and crisis that punctuated their lives. For the mothers in this study, habits like smoking were experienced less as a lifestyle choice and more as a life compromise, taken, in full knowledge of the health risks, to protect the welfare of the family.

Acknowledgements

The survey of mothers was funded by the Department of Health. The views expressed, however, are those of the author alone.

Notes

1 South Asian mothers were not included in the survey because of their low levels of smoking prevalence. The sampling criteria biased recruitment away from mothers and partners in non-manual occupations. As a result, the sample of claimant mothers may be more disadvantaged than the general population of mothers with young children dependent on income support. The high proportion of mothers in rented housing suggests that this is the case. However, low levels of owner-occupation also reflect the age profile of the sample and other measures, including household ownership of a car and a telephone, indicate living standards in line with national statistics for low-income households/households without an economically active head (Office of Population Censuses and Surveys 1991, 1994).

2 Recruitment to the original survey was stratified by smoking status, to yield a sample in which 50 per cent of the mothers were smokers. The smoking prevalence rate in the population from which the sample was drawn was 44 per cent. In order to ensure the representativeness of the sample of mothers on income support, smokers were randomly excluded from the original sample to produce a sample with an overall prevalence rate of 44 per cent prior to the identification of mothers on income support.

References

Cox, B.D. (ed.) (1987) *The Health and Lifestyle Survey*, London: Health Promotion Research Trust.

Department of Social Security (1994) *Social Security Statistics 1994*, London: HMSO.

Graham, H. (1993) *When Life's A Drag: Women, Smoking and Disadvantage*, London: HMSO

Lewis, J. (1980) *The Politics of Motherhood: Child and Maternal Welfare*, London: Croom Helm.

Office of Population Censuses and Surveys (1991) *1989 General Household Survey*, London: HMSO.

—— (1994) *1992 General Household Survey*, London: HMSO.

Smith, D.F. and Nicholson, M. (1992) 'Poverty and ill health: controversies past and present', *Proceedings of the Royal College of Physicians* 22: 190–9.

29 The body in consumer society*

Mike Featherstone

While the body incorporates fixed capacities such as height and bone structure, the tendency within consumer culture is for ascribed bodily qualities to become regarded as plastic – with effort and 'body work' individuals are persuaded that they can achieve a certain desired appearance. Advertising, feature articles and advice columns in magazines and newspapers ask individuals to assume self-responsibility for the way they look. This becomes important not just in the first flush of adolescence and early adulthood, for notions of 'natural' bodily deterioration and the bodily betrayals that accompany ageing become interpreted as signs of moral laxitude (Hepworth and Featherstone 1982). The wrinkles, sagging flesh, tendency towards middle age spread, hair loss etc, which accompany ageing should be combatted by energetic body maintenance on the part of the individual – with help from the cosmetic, beauty, fitness and leisure industries.

The perception of the body within consumer culture is dominated by the existence of a vast array of visual images. Indeed the inner logic of consumer culture depends upon the cultivation of an insatiable appetite to consume images. The production of images to stimulate sales on a societal level is echoed by the individual production of images through photography (Sontag 1978). Christopher Lasch (1979, p. 47) has noted the profound effect of photography on the perception of social life:

'Cameras and recording machines not only transcribe experience but alter its quality, giving to much of modern life the character of an enormous echo chamber, a hall of mirrors. Life presents itself as a succession of images, of electronic signals, of impressions recorded and reproduced by means of photography, motion pictures, television and sophisticated recording devices. Modern life is so thoroughly mediated by electronic images that we cannot help responding to others as if their actions – and our own – were being recorded and simultaneously transmitted to an unseen audience or stored up for close scrutiny at some later time'.

*This is an extract from Featherstone, M. 'The body in consumer society', *Theory, Culture and Society*, vol. 1, no. 2, pp. 18–33, 1982.

Day-to-day awareness of the current state of one's appearance is sharpened by comparison, with one's own past photographic images as well as with the idealised images of the human body which proliferate in advertising and the visual media. Images invite comparisons they are constant reminders of what we are and might with effort yet become. The desire for one's own body also becomes catered for with one of the effects of the new camera technology (instant photographs, video tapes) being to further private narcisstic uses.[1] Women are of course most clearly trapped in the narcissistic, self-surveillance world of images, for apart from being accorded the major responsibility in organising the purchase and consumption of commodities their bodies are used symbolically in advertisements (Winship 1980; Pollack 1977). The cosmetic and fashion industries are eager to redress this imbalance and promote men alongside women to enjoy the dubious equality of consumers in the market place (Winter and Robert 1980).

Images make individuals more conscious of external appearance, bodily presentation and 'the look'. The motion picture industry has since the early days of consumer culture been one of the major creators and purveyors of images. In this context it is interesting to note that Bela Balázs speculated in the early 1920s that film was transforming the emotional life of twentieth century man by directing him away from words towards movement and gesture. A culture dominated by words tends to be intangible and abstract, and reduces the human body to a basic biological organism, whereas the new emphasis upon visual images drew attention to the appearance of the body, the clothing, demeanour and gesture (Kern 1975).

The Hollywood cinema helped to create new standards of appearance and bodily presentation, bringing home to a mass audience the importance of 'looking good'. Hollywood publicised the new consumer culture values and projected images of the glamorous celebrity lifestyle to a worldwide audience. The major studios carefully disciplined and packaged film stars for audience consumption.[2] To ensure that the stars conformed with the ideals of physical perfection new kinds of make-up, hair care, and techniques such as electrolysis, cosmetic surgery and toupees were created to remove imperfections. Mary Pickford who subjected herself to a rigorous daily cosmetic, exercise and dietary regime in the early 1920s, later branched out into the cosmetic industry.

Helena Rubinstein, who amassed a fortune of over 500 million dollars, capitalised on these trends by enthusiastically advocating beauty for the masses. She reassured women that there was nothing wrong with wanting to hold onto youth and formulated the consumer culture equation of youth= beauty=health. 'To preserve one's beauty is to preserve health and prolong life' (Rubinstein 1930). The new female ideal (epitomised by the flapper) was not without its critics; Cynthia White (1970) remarks that editorials in British women's magazines in the early 1920s were firmly against the use of make-up and lipstick but by the late 1920s they had capitulated and were for cosmetics – a decision not unrelated to the increasing amount of cosmetic advertising they carried. The 1920s was a crucial decade in the formulation of the new bodily ideal. By the end of the decade women, under the combined impact of the cosmetic, fashion and advertising industries, and Hollywood, had for the first time in large numbers put on rouge and lipstick, taken to short skirts, rayon stockings and had abandoned the corset for rubber 'weight-reducing' girdles (Allen 1931). The new Hollywood styles threatened to carry all before them and iron out regional and local differences. JB Priestley (1977) on his English Journey of 1933, while taking tea in a rural cafe in Lincolnshire, noted that the girls of the nearby tables had carefully modelled their appearance on their favourite film stars:

> 'Even twenty years ago girls of this kind would have looked quite different even from girls in the nearest large town; they would have had an unmistakable small town rustic air; but now they are almost indistinguishable from girls in a dozen different capitals, for they all have the same models, from Hollywood.'

The major impact of the cosmetic, fashion and advertising industries in the inter-war years was on women; only slow inroads were made in the field of male fashions and cosmetics (one of the most difficult taboos to break down), until the 1960s and 70s. Yet Hollywood did help to bring about changes in the male ideal in the 1920s: Douglas Fairbanks, the first international cinema superstar, famous for the feats of athleticism he performed in costume spectaculars, was marketed as a virility symbol and fitness fanatic. Like his wife, Mary Pickford, disciplined body maintenance and routines played a prominent role in his private life with his daily training schedule of wrestling, boxing, running and swimming as strenuously publicised as his screen career (Walker 1970).

Fairbanks, who celebrated the athletic adventurous outdoor life in his films, also helped to popularise the sun tan. Going against the established wisdom which held that the fashionable body must avoid the effects of the sun, lest it be associated with the tanned labouring body, he allowed his darkened face to appear in films and the popular press. Other celebrities followed suit and sunbathing, which had emerged in the 1890s in Germany as a form of treatment of the tubercular, now gained a wider cosmetic appeal alongside its claims for health: 'The skin of the average overclothed man is white, spotty and inelastic, the skin of a healthy man is brown, smooth and sleek', proclaimed an American article of 1929. The inter-war years also saw the transformation of the beach into a place where one gained a suntan – the hallmark of a successful holiday. For the first time sunbathing on the beach brought together large numbers of people in varying degrees of undress, legitimating the public display of the body.

From its early days the publicity machine of Hollywood has catered for and generated a great deal of interest in the 'backstage' areas, the private lives of the stars, their beauty tips, exercise and diet regimes.[3] The Hollywood fan magazines of the 1920s and 1930s 'indoctrinated their true believers with the notions that women were beautiful, men were manly, crime didn't pay, lovers lived happily ever after time after time, and Lana Turner was discovered eating a sundae at Schwab's Drug Store' (Levin 1970, p. 7). Magazines such as *Photoplay*, *Silver Screen*, *Screen Book*, *Modern Screen* and *Motion Picture* as well as publicising the 'secrets of the stars' also offered readers the chance of self-improvement with advertisements claiming to provide remedies for acne, over-sized busts, under-sized busts, fatness etc. In the early days publicity stills of the stars were re-touched to eliminate blemishes in the actor's or actress' appearance, increasingly this work became unnecessary through the effort stars put into maintaining and enhancing their appearance: in effect they were able to become what they seemed. Hollywood stars began to rely less on aids and supports to effect a given appearance, rather they carefully achieved the appearance of the 'body natural'. Body supports such as the corset (later to reemerge as the naughty basque – a titillating body packaging aid for sexual fun and games) found less advocates in a culture which endorsed the exposure of the body on the beach and the wearing of casual leisure clothing. Increasingly exercise was presented as a healthy means of strengthening the body's natural support system (Hornibrook 1924), a technique which would enable the body to pass muster under the close gaze of the camera.

Body maintenance

"Stay young, stay beautiful, live longer. These are the catch phrases of today's hard living society . . . While the secret of longer life is still a long way off, many people are searching for a short cut – through health foods, yoga, gardening. Grab your survival kit and live longer."

The Sun

Body maintenance cannot of course be claimed as a novel creation of consumer culture. In traditional societies, religious communities such as monasteries demanded ascetic routines with an emphasis upon exercise and dietary control (Turner 1982). The adoption of ascetic regimes usually meant, however, that the body was subordinated to 'higher' spiritual ends. The dominant ethos of Christianity was to denigrate and repress the human body. Jesuits were taught on entering the order to accept Ignatius Loyola's maxim *Perinde ac cadavar* (henceforth as a corpse) (Benthall 1976, p. 69). The Christian tradition glorified an aesthetics of the soul not the body. Ascetic regimes would release the spirit and subdue the sexual side of the body. Within consumer culture on the other hand sexual experts proclaim that dietary control and exercise will enhance sexual prowess; exercise and sexuality are blurred together through neologisms such as "sexercise" and "exersex". The shame in the naked body gradually gave way under the persistent critique of sexual experts and commercial interests. To enjoy heightened pleasure individuals have not only to consult the sexual manual and resort to a growing range of pills, aids and devices, they must look good too. Self-surveillance through taking instant pictures and video-tapes celebrated sexual aesthetics: the naked body or the body packaged in erotic sexual leisure-wear could be recorded as proof of the achievement of a desired effect (Hepworth and Featherstone 1982).

The term 'body maintenance' indicates the popularity of the machine metaphor for the body. Like cars and other consumer goods, bodies require servicing, regular care and attention to preserve maximum efficiency.[4] As the consumption of goods increases, the time required for care and maintenance increases, and the same instrumental rational orientation adopted towards goods is turned inwards onto the body. The tendency to transform freetime into maintenance work imposes even greater demands on the individual and makes the monitoring of the current state of bodily performance essential if individuals are to get the most out of life: the hectic life increases the need for 'human servicing' (Linder 1970, p. 40).

Preventative medicine offers a similar message and through its offshoot, health education, demands constant vigilance on the part of the individual who has to be persuaded to assume responsibility for his health. Introducing the category 'self-inflicted illness', which results from body abuse (overeating, drinking, smoking, lack of exercise etc), health educationalists assert that individuals who conserve their bodies through dietary care and exercise will enjoy greater health and live longer. The calculation of the potential saving to state health services provides further grounds for castigating those who do not heed the new message as self-indulgent 'slobs' (Featherstone and Hepworth 1980, 1981; Hepworth and Featherstone 1982). In effect, the health education movement is trying to bring about a change in the moral climate so that individuals assume increasing self-responsibility for their health, body shape and appearance. To some extent, this can be seen as building on and accentuating self-help tendencies which were present within the Victorian middle class whose preoccupation with health matters lead them to diet, take pills, take up athletics etc (Haly 1979). Yet however much health education-alists appeal to the rationality of self-preservation and offer the incentives of longevity and lowered risk of disease, their body maintenance messages are strongly influenced by the consumer culture idealisation of youth and the body beautiful. In the late 1970s, the British Health Education Council found that the most effective advertising message was to highlight the cosmetic rewards of fitness and dietary care. Health educationalists have little time for the health food crank or the fitness fanatic in their advertisements, these are discarded in favour of images of men and women who maximise, who get more out of life, who 'look good and feel good', who are more attractive and therefore socially acceptable. Within this logic, fitness and slimness become associated not only with energy, drive and vitality but worthiness as a person; likewise the body beautiful comes to be taken as a sign of prudence and prescience in health matters.

The popular media and commercial interests have found the 'looking good and feeling great' health education message to be a saleable commodity. Eager to endorse body maintenance as a part of the consumer lifestyle, popular newspapers like *The Sun* and *Mirror* in Britain pass on the message to a wider audience with frequent articles on slimming, exercise, health foods, and appearance. Centre-page spreads enable readers to calculate their degree of success or failure in meeting age/height/weight targets and how to complete questionnaires to work out their 'survival power'. Feature articles on the calorific value of different types of food complement centre-page spreads on the calorie burning power of different types of activity (running, sitting, walking, sleeping, kissing, sex etc), enabling the enterprising reader to draw up a daily calorific balance sheet to see if he or she can meet their designated target. In the last decade, there has also been a noticeable growth in the number of specialist magazines on jogging, running, health foods, exercise, and especially slimming. Self-help books on body maintenance also sell well: in December 1981 four out of ten books on the US bestseller list were of the 'how to lose weight' variety. Common to the popular media treatment of body maintenance, be it from the popular press, specialist magazines of the 'Doctors Answers' type, advertisements for vitamins, slimming products or government health education propaganda, is the encouragement of self-surveillance of bodily health and appearance as well as the incentive of lifestyle benefits. Body maintenance is firmly established as a virtuous leisure time activity which will reap further lifestyle rewards resulting from an enhanced appearance: body maintenance in order to look good merges with the stylised images of looking good while maintaining the body. The images in the advertisements, popular press and health education pamphlets are of lithe, bright-eyed beautiful people, in varying states of nakedness, enjoying their body work. The fat are invariably portrayed as glum and downcast: joke figures, survivals from a bygone age.

One of the noticeable features of the 20th century, according to Theodore Zeldin (1977, p. 440), has been the triumph of the thin woman over the fat woman. It can be added that in the second half of the 20th century this ideal is becoming firmly established for men too, with the last bastions of corpulence amongst the working class now under siege. As the slim form becomes mandatory, almost every conceivable consumer product is discovered to have slimming properties. In 1931, the manufacturers of Lucky Strike cigarettes spent 19 million dollars on advertising and successfully convinced many women that smoking was a vital aid to dieting (Susman 1973, p. 132). Today grapefruit juice, disco dancing, plankton and sex are marketed with similar conviction. The beauty industry now offers 'shapeovers' ('look 10 pounds slimmer without dieting')[5] to accompany 'makeovers' as an essential part of every woman's cosmetic repertoire.

Within consumer culture slimness has become associated with health and the health educational message that being overweight is a health risk has become absorbed into the conventional wisdom. Yet a good deal of the 'advice' that abounds in the media and advertisements is clearly of a pseudo-scientific nature. Rubin Andres has recently conducted an extensive review of a number of slimming studies and concluded that the overweight actually live longer. The age/height/weight charts originally constructed by insurance companies, which hang in doctors surgeries and are publicised in the popular media, are inaccurate – in some cases as much as a stone out. Andres' conclusion that slimness has little to do with health merely confirms those reached by earlier researchers such as Bruch (1957) and Beller (1977) and may be destined to have a similar lack of impact.

Women of course are well aware that the major reason for dieting is cosmetic and that 'looking good' not only becomes necessary to achieve social acceptability but can become the key to a more exciting lifestyle. As one woman remarked in a slimming magazine article: 'Being overweight was, for me, like living with the brakes on. And I *hated* being held back.' The lifestyle benefits are played up in slimming magazines and the popular press: not only do successful slimmers get more admiring glances, they feel more attractive and are confident to go out more, take up new exciting hobbies and live out their version of the Martini people lifestyle (Hepworth and Featherstone 1982).

Like slimming, jogging provides further insight into the transvaluation of use within consumer culture: everything has to be good for something else and the range of alleged benefits multiplies endlessly. Apart from reducing the chance of coronary heart disease, it is claimed jogging helps to cure impotence, increase confidence, psychological well-being, and puts 'you in control of your body'. Jogging has also been claimed to result in prolonged cosmetic benefits – improving posture, reducing stomach sag, helping to burn off excessive fat (Hepworth and Featherstone 1982, p. 107). The notion of running for running's sake, purposiveness without purpose, a sensuous experience in harmony with embodied and physical nature, is completely submerged amidst the welter of benefits called up by the market and health experts (Featherstone and Hepworth 1982).

The instrumental strategies which body maintenance demands of the individual resonate with deep-seated features of consumer culture which encourage individuals to negotiate their social relationships and approach their free time activities with a calculating frame of mind. Self-preservation depends upon the preservation of the body within a culture in which the body is the passport to all that is good in life. Health, youth, beauty, sex, fitness are the positive attributes which body care can achieve and preserve. With appearance being taken as a reflex of the self the penalties of bodily neglect are a lowering of one's acceptability as a person, as well as an indication of laziness, low self-esteem and even moral failure. Within consumer culture it is hardly surprising that ageing and death are viewed so negatively – they are unwelcome reminders of the inevitable decay and defeat that are in store, even for the most vigilant of individuals. The secularisation of the body has resulted in the eclipse of the traditional religious purpose of the body in which it was regarded as a transitory vehicle, a means to higher spiritual ends. Today, pain, suffering and death are seen as unwelcome intrusions in the midst of a happy life (Ariès 1974) and the consumer culture imagery has decreed that life can and should be everlastingly happy. Amidst images of comfort, fulfilment and cleanliness the unpleasant odours and sights surrounding death become intolerable: 'the dirty death' (Ariès 1981, p. 568) has to be hidden away.

Notes

* I would like to thank John Alt, Josef Bleicher and Mike Hepworth for comments on the earlier draft of this paper. Many of the ideas in this paper draw on my joint work with Mike Hepworth.
1 One British daily newspaper in 1981 referred to a firm which specialised in a home videotape service for couples. They would devise a plot and photograph the couple engaged in sex. The tape could then be played back at their leisure and would serve as a momento in old age of how they once performed.
2 The star system was not the invention of Hollywood. Hess and Nochlin (1973) remark that it originated in the 1890s with the theatrical publicity picture (e.g. Toulouse-Lautrec). The image of the star was reduced to a salient gesture on property (e.g. Sarah Bernhardt's tresses). The more these attributes became fixed in the public's mind, the more the star's actual appearance tended to become stylised and rigid.
3 Today it is not only the secrets of the stars but those of politicians too which cause interest. Public relations experts take the media on tours of politicians backstage areas to divulge the body maintenance routines which produce the energy, vitality, health and zest-for-life of politician-celebrities such as Ford, Carter, Reagan and Thatcher.
4 See for example O. Gillie (1978) *The Sunday Times Book of Body Maintenance*, Diagram Group (1977) *Man's Body: An Owner's Manual*.
5. The headline of a double page spread in the *News of the World* magazine *Sunday*, in January 1982. The text, surrounding a picture of a young woman in a leotard smiling as she exercised, referred to exercises devised by Adrian Arpel, 'America's queen of self-improvement', the 'boss of her own international cosmetics business' who claimed 'anyone can shed ten pounds and ten years without a diet or facelift'.

References

Allen, P.L. (1931) *Only Yesterday*, Volume 1, Harmondsworth: Penguin.
Ariès, P. (1974) *Western Attitudes Towards Death*, Johns Hopkins UP.
Ariès, P. (1981) *The Hour of Our Death*, New York: Knopf.
Beller, A.S. (1977) *Fat and Thin: A Natural History of Obesity*, New York: Farrar, Strauss & Giroux.
Benthall, J. (1976) *The Body Electric: Patterns of Western Industrial Culture*, London: Thames and Hudson.
Bruch, H. (1957) *The Importance of Overweight*, New York: W. Norton.
Diagram Group (1977) *Man's Body: An Owner's Manual*, London: Corgi.
Featherstone, M. and Hepworth, M. (1980) 'Changing Images of Middle Age', in M. Johnson (ed.) *Transitions in Middle and Later Life*, London: British Society of Gerontology.
Featherstone, M. and Hepworth, M. (1981) 'Images de la maturité', *Gerontologie*, Dec.
Featherstone, M. and Hepworth, M. (1982) 'Ageing and Inequality: Consumer Culture and the New Middle Age' in D. Robbins et al. (eds) *Rethinking Social Inequality*, Gower P.

Gillie, O. (1978) *The Sunday Times Book of Body Maintenance*, London: Joseph.

Haly, B. (1979) *The Healthy Body and Victorian Culture*, Cambridge: Harvard UP.

Hepworth, M. and Featherstone, M. (1982) *Surviving Middle Age*, Oxford: B. Blackwell.

Hess, T.B. and Nochlin, N. (1973) *Woman as Sex Object*, London: Allen Lane.

Hornibrook, F.A. (1924) *The Cult of the Abdomen: The Cure of Obesity and Constipation*, London: Heinemann.

Kern, S. (1975) *Anatomy and Destiny: A Cultural History of the Human Body*, Bobbs-Merrill.

Lasch, C. (1979) *The Culture of Narcissism*, New York: Norton.

Levin, M. (1970) *Hollywood and the Great Fan Magazines*, London: Ian Allen.

Linder, S.B. (1970) *The Harried Leisure Class*, New York: Columbia UP.

Pollack, G. (1977) 'What's Wrong With Images of Women?' *Screen Education*, 24, 1.

Priestley, J.B. (1977) *English Journey* (orig. 1934), Harmondsworth: Penguin.

Rubinstein, H. (1930) *The Art of Feminine Beauty*, New York: Liveright.

Sontag, S. (1978) *On Photography*, London: Allen Lane.

Susman, W. (1973) *Culture and Commitment 1929–1945*, New York: Braziller.

Turner, B.S. (1982) 'The Discourse of Diet', *Theory, Culture and Society*, 1, 1.

Walker, A. (1970) *Stardom: The Hollywood Phenomenon*, New York: Stein and Day.

White, C.L. (1970) *Women's Magazines 1693–1968*, London: Joseph.

Winter, M.F. and Robert, E.R. (1980) 'Male Domination, Late Capitalism and the Growth of Instrumental Reason', *Berkeley Journal of Sociology*.

Winship, J. (1980) 'Sexuality for Sale', in S. Hall, D. Hobson, A. Lowe and P. Willis (eds) *Culture, Media, Language*, London: Hutchinson.

Zeldin, T. (1977) *France 1848–1945, Volume 2: Intellect, Taste and Anxiety*, Oxford, Oxford UP.

30 Containing the body*

Wendy Seymour

Continence

The chapter will draw on data from an empirical study of twenty-four people with varying degrees of bodily paralysis resulting from a range of serious conditions, material which is developed more fully in a recently released publication (Seymour 1998). Most of the informants have sustained damage to their spinal cord. The loss of muscle power associated with these conditions is usually obvious but few people realise that deep and superficial sensation, vasomotor control, bladder and bowel control and sexual function may also be lost. Since spinal cord damage is permanent, rehabilitation is directed towards utilising the remaining intact functions and developing strategies for maintaining essential bodily functions. Care of the bladder and the bowel must become obsessional, since neglect of these vital parts of the body can have extremely serious clinical consequences (Jones & Davidson 1988, p. 109). While the loss of bowel and bladder control associated with these conditions provides dramatic examples of faecal and urinary incontinence, the broader issue of bodily continence involves a range of fluids and substances which engage with the body in a variety of ways.

The informants graphically describe the experience of living in a leaking body. Anthony says, 'You can't control when you urinate, nor do you know when you are using your bowels. It is very scary, and very threatening. The need to protect yourself means that you do not open up to people.' Joy claims that 'You lose all your modesty – you know, shitting and urinating in front of people and stuff like that. It really hurts your pride.' Ken says

> One of the most demeaning and belittling things is not having control over your bowels. It creates enormous feelings of powerlessness. I was having accidents daily, more than daily. Every time I did anything physical, my bowels would move, not much sometimes, but enough to create a helluva mess and a smell.

*This is an extract from a chapter first published in Petersen, A. and Waddell, C. (eds) (1998) *Health Matters: A Sociology of Illness, Prevention and Care*, Allen & Unwin/Open University Press, pp. 156–68.

Frances describes her early experiences as 'excruciating'. 'I was mortified every time it happened. I hated the fact that people had to come to change the sheets. It was just awful. I can remember that I was smelly, I was just vile, the gas that was coming from me was just terrible.' Bridget, too, is unequivocal that the loss of bladder and bowel function was the worst aspect of her disability, 'I had to wear these big nappies at first. With the suppositories you flood all over the toilet. It was a real hassle.' Although Mark's injury was many years ago he still remembers 'the mess, you know, shitting myself, having accidents, and that went on for quite a number of years after I left the unit'.

Unlike babies in the animal kingdom, the human baby is born with an 'unfinished' body (Gehlen 1988, p. 4). The newborn baby cannot fend for itself but must depend on others to attend to its nourishment, shelter and the management of sleep and bodily excretions. Gradually infants learn to control aspects of their bodies, and attend to their own needs. The child's internal bodily processes are regulated as well as the child's behaviour, appearance and view of the world. Civilisation is, thus, an ongoing process of body taming. Human bodies have to be trained, manipulated, cajoled, coaxed, organised and disciplined in order to fit into society (Elias 1978). Civilised life depends on the successful presenting, monitoring and interpreting of bodies; culture is a product of the complex interweaving of the body and society. The body is neither a product of biology nor a product of society. The body is 'simultaneously, conjointly and concurrently socially and organically founded' (Turner 1992, p. 7). Although society plays a critical role in the constitution of the body, it is the body which may present society with its potentiality and with its most formidable resistance.

Socialisation

Toilet training is a potent vehicle for introducing a child to the concept of shame (Lawler 1991, p. 137). Civilising the bladder and bowel to conform to social rules about the timing and placement of bodily wastes involves a systematic process of encouraging the baby to take on the parent's attitudes, and through the parent, the values of the wider social group to which the parent belongs, in relation to these activities (Turner 1987, p. 85). This process is achieved through orthodox behaviour modification strategies where children are rewarded for behaving in a way that conforms to their parents' values, and punished when they do not.

The concept of modesty – the acknowledgement of the need to privatise the 'private parts' of the body (Elias 1978, pp. 31–32) – has developed alongside the processes designed to civilise the body. The sequestering of particular parts and functions of the body that are 'best not talked about' makes people vulnerable to embarrassment and shame (Elias 1978, p. 190).

A well-socialised adult understands the need to protect the sensibilities of others from untoward sights, sounds and smells that may emanate from the body. Public health messages are based on similar imperatives (Petersen &

Lupton 1996). A responsible citizen must work on their own body in order to defend it against moral, bacteriological and physical invasion. At the same time the citizen must assume responsibility for ensuring that these bodily regimens are sufficiently rigorous to protect others from contamination. In the contemporary era a citizen is expected to assume onerous responsibilities for monitoring, discipling and controlling their body. But how much control does an individual have over their body in a context of disease, damage and rapidly escalating global risk? (Beck 1992; Petersen & Lupton 1996).

Disease and illness have long been imbued with moral implications (Turner 1996, p. 97). Contemporary public health is still a moral enterprise (Petersen & Lupton 1996): the 'new' public health remains embedded within a discourse which underlines the responsibilities and duties that individuals should assume in relation to their bodies in return for the privilege of citizenship. Health economics are played out in a multitude of sites, but within the context of modern hospital management, the insurance industry and the new public health we are witnessing an increasingly direct linkage between individual behaviours and disease or trauma. While victim blaming is by no means a new invention, the recent emergence of the concept of the 'entrepreneurial self' – the self who is expected to live life in a prudent and calculating way, well informed and mindful of the risks to the body – is clearly a product of the retreat from the welfare state and reliance on markets to regulate the economy (Petersen & Lupton 1996, p. xiii).

In this context people who have sustained damage to their bodies through trauma or accidents involving alcohol or drug usage, travelling at high speeds or risk-taking behaviours such as diving into shallow water or hang-gliding are particularly susceptible to implications of irresponsibility. They may feel a heightened sense of obligation to manage their anarchic body in a manner which will cause as little further distress to others as possible. Successful body management, especially in the area of bodily continence, will provide evidence of a renewed sense of responsibility and commitment to core social values.

Continence then, can be seen as the conquest of the body by society, a victory which is reinforced by the context of privacy, modesty, propriety and shame within which the bodily activities take place. The victory, however, is always tentative. Our anxieties about continence reflect our perpetual fear that the body may defy its years of careful socialisation and training and reassert its pre-civilised nature. The unregulated permeability of bodily fluids represents a serious source of danger and pollution (Butler 1990, p. 132). Conditions or practices which refocus attention to particular areas of the body, or redefine the expectations of activities previously taken for granted are distressing because they threaten to disrupt the stability of the body and question our status as properly civilised, responsible citizens.

Formal bladder and bowel retraining in rehabilitation units aims to condition the bladder and the bowel to empty at convenient times and in convenient places, a process not unlike the toilet training procedures of childhood. A young child learns to be ashamed as part of the social process of toilet training. While the sense of 'feeling like a baby' sums up the experiences of most of the informants, these people have well established attitudes towards bodily continence. Their sense of shame is fully developed. To attempt to reconcile such feelings about oneself with the inexorable reality of incontinence in the face of other people's revulsion to bodily products is a constant attack on the embodied self.

Although Mary claims that 'bladder problems are endless' she continues, more forcefully, to say:

> But I don't think that there is a word bad enough to describe the problems associated with the bowel. Bladder training is a euphemism. It doesn't train your bladder at all, it just means that you beat your bladder to it. As far as my bowels are concerned, I go once a day. Something may or may not happen, and it's a revolting process. I've been down the suppository track. I have ended up having to do it with a gloved hand, what's called 'manual removal'. In my case it's a very messy occupation, and it prevents me going away to stay overnight. What on earth would I do if I found myself with a toilet that is unsuitable, and I made an awful mess that I'd have to clean up?

Rosemary has an ileostomy bag for urinary elimination; faecal material, though, must be manually removed from her bowel. Her mother has done this for her all her life, but as Rosemary says, 'Now I am getting older I should try to do this for myself'. Alister claims that he was not distressed by the rigorous, formal program of bladder and bowel management that is central to spinal injury rehabilitation. He was able to see the catheterisation and suppositories as 'practical measures which just had to be done. Well you have no choice. You either do it or you don't cope.' Jenny is less phlegmatic. 'With the lack of bladder control, you were constantly having to have your sheets changed – every few hours, day and night. I found all of that a real intrusion. There were lots and lots of jokes, "Oh you're wet again", and "Didn't your mother toilet train you?", or whatever.' Alister's attitude towards this aspect of rehabilitation is rare; most of the men and women perceive the practices and implications arising from this loss as a destructive incursion into their embodied selves, and a recurring attack on their bodily integrity and self-esteem throughout their lives.

The perineum may be a relatively small area of the body, but it contains a concentration of bodily openings. Danger is focused in this area because of the pathway these orifices offer between the body and the outside world. Semen, vaginal secretions, faeces, urine and blood pass from the body: bacteriological, physical and moral invaders may enter the body through these external portals. If the body provides a schema for society as Mary Douglas suggests (1966), it is not hard to see how this part of the body is invested with inordinate importance. Sex and excretion are thus highly dangerous activities. Our ideas of cleanliness and purity are closely aligned with these activities.

It is in this small, but highly defended part of the body where society may be most threatened. In no other part of the body is the tension so tightly drawn. While few able-bodied men and women are unaware of the volatile nature of the perineal area, most people develop a range of strategies to divert themselves and the attentions of others from this dangerous territory. The lifelong preoccupation with bodily eliminations and relentless concentration of energy and attention to the genital area are the issues to which people with body paralyses must attend. Yet this context of leaking fluids and permeable boundaries may also be a site of contestation and new possibilities.

For a considerable time, however, most of the informants expressed profound distress at what they termed the 'abnormality' of their situation. As George says, 'the worst impact of bowel and bladder loss is the abnormality of it all'. For several years he didn't go anywhere 'because it was just too hard'. He now manages all the aspects of bowel and bladder function himself. Joy, too, feels this loss most profoundly. 'I miss the feeling of wanting to go to the toilet, you know, you miss things like that, the feeling of a full bladder or just going to the toilet. I dream about it all the time. In my dreams it's so real, it feels like it's real.' Because some of the sensory nerves were spared in Anthony's spinal injury, the retraining program was more likely to be successful. He speaks of 'the great joy and excitement I had when I started to be able to go to the toilet and use my bowels again – the sensation and the feeling!' The elation at achieving what seem such mundane goals after two years of effort highlights the dramatic impact of this aspect of bodily damage.

Eating and drinking are major preoccupations of our lives. While biomedicine sees these activities as fundamental to the survival of the human organism and as risk factors in some diseases, recent developments in the sociology of food and consumption (Crotty 1995; Falk 1994; Lupton, 1996; Mennell et al. 1992; Turner 1992, ch. 6) have expanded such restrictive notions. When we eat and drink we engage in a complex range of personal and social acts which may have little overt connection with survival or disease prevention. Clearly the rationalisation of eating practices and the growth of dietary sciences epitomise Foucault's connection between the body, knowledge and power (Turner 1992, p. 192), yet food and drink are also associated with appetites, desires, comforts, satisfactions, sexualities and other bodily pleasures which have far less rational connotations.

Rehabilitation of the leaky body involves strict adherence to a range of bodily regimens. Desires and appetites for food and drink must be modified in order to discipline the body and regulate its fluids. The body is subdued by means of painstaking experimentation and monitoring of bodily processes. It is only by constant surveillance of the body and monitoring of its fluids that the chaotic body can be restored to a semblance of order, a fragile truce.

Pam describes the extensive program of bodily surveillance in which she engaged before she developed some strategies for control. She says, 'I went through a process of measuring what I drank. I used to sit on the portable commode by the hour just finding out how long it took to come through and then measure it.' Pam claims that it took about six months after she returned home from the rehabilitation unit to develop some confidence in her bladder, although she still has accidents. Many years later she still monitors her intake very carefully, but social functions, sickness and even climatic variations can threaten this uneasy equilibrium.

Not surprisingly, this process encourages the men and women in the study to reconceptualise their bodies in terms of a well-integrated, but simple, hydraulic system of pipes, plumbing, substances and fluids (Turner 1992, p. 184). Inputs are carefully manipulated to ensure satisfactory outputs. Constant attention must be given to the timing and nature of the food and drink taken into their bodies in order to minimise the possibility of inopportune leakage. The body is seen as a machine that requires continual surveillance for optimal performance, and in order to operate in a manner which will not offend others. Dietary management, careful living and regular habits serve to produce a well-contained body which will not threaten society by its anarchic activities. Anxieties associated with the uncontrolled leakage of bodily fluids are reassured by evidence of strict observation of bodily regimens associated with the government of the body (Turner 1992, p. 192). Clearly these bodies have come to epitomise the notion of the mechanical body which lies at the heart of biomedicine.

Although many of the informants have been successful in devising ways to manage their wayward bladders and bowels to fit their own lifestyles, most live with a heightened sense of the risks involved in failing to balance the tensions between bodily input and output. The necessity to continually monitor these activities compromises the spontaneity and freedom of choice we associate with eating and drinking. While such practices will result in a degree of predictability for many people, this regulation threatens to subordinate the body. Rigorous self-surveillance, discipline and deference to regimens of diet and timetables of bodily evacuation must surely challenge the embodied self. But just as appetite and sexuality are major threats to the aestheticism which underpins religious vocation (Turner 1992, p. 178), so too are appetites and sexualities key areas for subversion of the regulated body. While dietary regimes may subdue the body, the desire and appetite for food may subvert this regulation.

References

Beck, U. 1992 *Risk Society: Towards a New Modernity* Sage, London.

Butler, J. 1990 *Gender Trouble: Feminism and the Subversion of Identity,* Routledge, London.

Crotty, P. 1995 *Good Nutrition? Fact and Fashion in Dietary Advice,* Allen & Unwin, Sydney.

Douglas, M. 1966 *Purity and Danger: An Analysis of the Concepts of Pollution and Taboo,* Routledge & Kegan Paul, UK.

Elias, N. 1978 *The Civilizing Process: Vol. 1: The History of Manners,* Urizen books, New York.

Falk, P. 1994 *The Consuming Body*, Sage, London.

Gehlen, A. 1988 *Man. His Nature and Place in the World*, trans. C. McMillan & K. Pillemer, Columbia University Press, New York.

Jones, G. & Davidson, J. 1988 'How spinal cord paralysis affects body image' in *Altered Body Image – The Nurse's Role,* ed. M. Salter, John Wiley & Sons Ltd, Guildford.

Lawler, J. 1991 *Behind the Screens: Nursing, Somology, and the Problem of the Body,* Churchill Livingstone, Melbourne.

Lupton, D. 1996 *Food, the Body and the Self,* Sage, London.

Mennell, S., Murcott, A. & van Otterloo, A. 1992 *The Sociology of Food: Eating, Diet and Culture*, Sage, London.

Petersen, A. & Lupton, D. 1996 *The New Public Health: Health and Self in the Age of Risk,* Allen & Unwin, Sydney.

Seymour, W. 1998 *Remaking the Body: Rehabilitation and Change,* Allen & Unwin, Sydney.

Turner, B. 1987 *Medical Power and Social Knowledge*, Sage, London.

—— 1992 *Regulating Bodies: Essays in Medical Sociology*, Routledge, London.

—— 1996 *The Body & Society: Explorations in Social Theory*, 2nd edn, Sage, London.

31 A good enough death*

Beverley McNamara

Dying is not often discussed in the context of health, and indeed each could be viewed as the antithesis of the other. However, 'health' and 'dying' are not discrete states, and the degree of relativity between the two varies for philosophical as well as practical reasons. A good death which implies a degree of quality and dignity in the dying process is more closely aligned to the concept of health than a 'good enough' death or even a 'bad' death. Also, the ageing population in advanced industrialised societies[1] has meant that the gradual decline of health to a state of ill health and further to a state of dying may be a protracted stage of a person's life. Much of what happens to a person during this time of failing health and approaching death will be determined by the pathology of their disease as well as their physical strength and personal resolve. Yet individual characteristics cannot fully explain the circumstances of each person's journey towards death. Cultural responses to dying and death as well as broader social structures frame the experience of each individual.

There are two distinct things that happen to the terminally ill person: the death of the body and the 'passing' of the person (Cassell 1975, p. 45). Dying, therefore, is not simply a biological fact, but a social process; and death, not a moment in time, but a social phenomenon. The meanings of both dying and death are not invariant (Gavin 1995, p. 75); they are constructed differently over time and in different cultural contexts (Aries 1974; Metcalfe & Huntington 1991). For terminally ill people, therefore, it is not just their health or ill health that matters, but the manner in which dying and death is understood when and where their life ends. In this chapter I will explore some of the issues that arise in the time before death, when terminally ill people, together with their families and health professional carers, negotiate the circumstances of dying. While most of the discussion is relevant to all terminally ill people, I will illustrate theoretical perspectives with examples drawn from my ethnographic fieldwork in Australian hospices and palliative

*This is a chapter that was first published in Petersen, A. and Waddell, C. (eds) (1998) *Health Matters: A Sociology of Illness, Prevention and Care*, Allen & Unwin/Open University Press, pp. 169–84.

care services. Most people who use these services suffer from cancer, though palliative care is now becoming increasingly more available to people with other non-malignant diseases.

The terminally ill person's experience, particularly their quality of life, will be influenced largely by their ability to participate in decisions that are made about them in the last days of their life. These decisions might relate to life-prolonging medical treatments, to issues of pain control and the degree to which the dying person is conscious, or even to the place and the time of death. Decision-making at the end of life seems particularly important in the current climate of patient 'empowerment' and individual responsibility. Individualism, however, often becomes more a rhetorical construct than an observable and effectual reality when dying people, exhausted by illness and grief, negotiate with varying degrees of ability and support, the circumstances of their own deaths. How then can we understand death to be good; or are most deaths simply 'good enough'? I propose five inter-related factors which inform the manner in which people die in advanced industrialised societies. These are: (1) cultural constructions of individualism; (2) the terminally ill person's altered conceptions of self and their capacity for autonomous decision-making; (3) social location and structural constraints; (4) biomedical culture; and (5) local moral culture. These five factors influence the extent to which each person's dying and ultimate death can be understood as 'good' or 'good enough'.

Death: 'good' or 'good enough' in hospice?

The Good Death is an idealised concept, particularly in the context of a hospice and palliative care setting, where terminally ill people who have stopped curative treatments are cared for in a supportive environment. Good death, which literally means euthanasia (Veatch 1976), has here been reconstructed to mean a process where the terminally ill person, their family, and the health professional team share a mutual acceptance of the terminally ill person's approaching death and engage in shared decision-making. Above all, this manner of dying is said to be dignified and peaceful. Many factors impinge upon the realisation of this ideal which I have detailed elsewhere (McNamara et al. 1994, 1995) but for the purposes of the discussion in this chapter it is important to note that Good Deaths can only happen if the dying person, the family and the health professionals all agree with what is happening in the time before death. It is also significant that when people are dying from cancer and other chronic illnesses they require substantial medical and nursing care. The stage upon which these dramas unfold therefore, is most significantly that of medicine.

While the area of hospice and palliative care has traditionally been viewed as relatively marginal to mainstream medicine, it still tends to be part of the vast cultural system of biomedicine. The hospice–palliative model of care, based upon the broader social movement of hospice evident in North America and Britain, arose in response to the inappropriate, technological and clinical approach to dying people that was evident in the 1960s and 1970s. There has been a large degree of integration of the palliative care model into the mainstream of medical care, but this model still continues to serve as a symbolic critique of how dying people are managed in other terminal care settings. Yet paradoxically, hospice and palliative care is dependent on the structural and ritual foundations of medicine and the national health care system. Such tension forms a backdrop for the ideological framework of hospice and palliative care which focuses on the needs and wishes of the individual patient and their close social circle.

Many health professionals who work within the area of hospice and palliative care have often expressed reservations about the ideal of a Good Death, considering either open discussion concerning death or shared decision-making to be problematic. An alternative way of looking at the interaction that takes place in the time before death is to propose the idea of a death that is 'good enough'. A 'good enough' death has been described by two prominent palliative care practitioners as a death 'as close as possible to the circumstances the person would have chosen' (Campbell 1990, p. 2) and 'a death with integrity, consistent with the life that person has led' (Komesaroff et al. 1995, p. 597). Both of these interpretations are consistent with the recent theoretical position that authority over dying should be invested in the individual. Closer examination of these seemingly humanistic and person-centred definitions, however, reveals that the focus on the individual can be empowering on one hand, yet on the other hand, it can act as a means to shift the locus of responsibility. A 'good enough' death does not happen through the individual conception of self in relation to what the dying person was or what they wanted, but to what they see themselves as being now and what they are able to decide upon now. Furthermore, the death is 'good enough' because it is close enough to individual wishes. The question arises: what factors constrain individual wishes? In order to understand the implications of a 'good enough' death it is necessary to trace the social and historical contexts of individualism in relation to medical care.

The individual's authority over dying

The concern with the authority of the individual over dying can be traced broadly to two trends: first, a societal preoccupation with individuality; and secondly, a growing dissatisfaction among the lay and professional communities with both the power and limitations of medicine. With regards to the first of these trends, Kellehear (1996, pp. 88–89) has noted that present attitudes towards death are 'forged from the material and social conditions of the baby-boomer generation'. He suggests that focusing on the individual has become a moral and ethical imperative. Moller (1990) contributes to this discussion by arguing that the technological development of modern society, with its associated bureaucratic rationality, has created an ideology of individualism.

Both Bauman (1992) and Elias (1985) have argued that the self-care policy of survival (individual concerns with health and fitness of the body) construes death as an individual event. Furthermore, they have commented on the increasing secularisation and privatisation of contemporary society. The group of people who gather around the bed of the dying person generally do not have a shared system of belief, be it religion, magic or science, to temper what Elias (1985) has called the loneliness of dying. The degree to which death has become taboo (Gorer 1965; Aries 1981) or sequestrated from public view (Mellor & Shilling 1993) within society is a contentious issue (Kellehear 1984; Walters 1991). However, there seems to be an agreement within the literature that the privatisation and subjectification of the experience of death 'results in the increased presence of considerations of death for individuals' (Mellor 1993, p. 12).

The second trend which has led to the re-examination of the authority of the individual over dying points to a critique which comes from both within and without the profession of medicine. Social scientists have been prominent in the discussion surrounding the use of technology as a means of unnecessarily prolonging life, delaying death or even engaging in a conquest of death (Parsons et al. 1972; Illich 1976; Lock 1996). It has been suggested that the medical model makes it difficult, if not impossible, to decide that any given person shall be allowed to die (Muller & Koenig 1988). Responding to these criticisms, Kelner and Bourgeault (1993) have suggested that health professionals must concede their professional autonomy and enter into a partnership with patients in end of life decision-making. In Chapter 18 of this volume, Kellehear traces the recent public expectation of control over dying to the rise of the New Public Health which has fostered empowering social forces for the individual.

This message of empowerment and the dissatisfaction of community members with the medicalisation of death, most evident in the social movement of hospice in North America and Britain, but also in popular media presentations, has influenced many members of the medical profession to varying degrees. North American surgeon Nuland, whose book *How We Die: Reflections on Life's Final Chapter* (1994) has gained a large popular readership in the English-speaking world, while critical of medical technology, cautions that inevitably the rescue credo of high technology medicine overrides personal choice. In the Australian context the message of community dissatisfaction with end of life treatments appears to have reached some medical practitioners:

Many health professionals believe that more people can have better deaths, that enough is known to make dying more tolerable for many of us, and that too many of today's problems rest with the attitudes of providers as much as with anything else.

(Baume 1993, p. 792)

A recent survey made clear that end of life treatment is 'significantly determined by an array of individual characteristics of the doctor and not solely by the nature of the medical problem'. However, it was also noted that, of the doctors surveyed, most believed that they adhere to patient and family wishes when they are known, providing the patient has not requested euthanasia (Waddell et al. 1996, p. 540).

The focus on the individual and that person's ability to be part of the discussions surrounding their dying has become a feature of the modern hospice–palliative model of care within Australia. Hunt, a doctor and pioneer in hospice and palliative care in South Australia writes the following:

> The principle of autonomy was neglected in terminal care before the development of hospice and palliative care – most patients were ill-informed of their situation, and they were submissive to medical paternalism. The palliative mode emphasised the importance of sensitively informing patients about their state of health and the treatment options available to them, and stressed the importance of patients being involved in decisions about their quality of life. The shift to the palliative mode, therefore, moved the power base in the relationship between health carers and patients, from professional domination to increased patient autonomy.
>
> (1994, p. 131)

Whether the principle of autonomy in terminal care can be traced solely to the development of hospice and palliative care is debatable given the social and historical contexts of both individuality in dying and death and the growing consumer dissatisfaction with all medical care. However, suffice to say this social movement both grew out of and further fuelled the impetus for patient autonomy in terminal care, which has now begun to reach beyond the bounds of hospice and palliative care. Nevertheless, it seems that in the discussion regarding patient autonomy there is an oversight which relates to the way in which 'individual' or 'self' is taken as *a priori* and not seen as relevant to the way decisions are made. Yet in the course of daily practice terminally ill people, their loved ones and health professionals are consistently confronted with conflicting understandings of individuality, self, personhood, autonomy, and so on.

Dying in advanced industrialised societies

So far in this chapter I have argued that the ability to participate in decision-making at the end of life had become a feature of 'modern' dying. Furthermore, participation and empowerment have become principal criteria in determining whether a person has a 'good' or 'good enough' death. As the Good Death is an idealised concept which is often unrealised, a 'good enough' death appears to be a far more workable definition with which to link participation in end of life decision-making. The following five inter-related factors inform the manner in which people die in advanced industrialised societies. They illustrate the degree to which cultural and individual responses, as well as broader social structures, frame the experience of each terminally ill person.

Social constructions of individualism

Just as dying and death are understood to mean different things at different times and places, the concept of individual or self is historically and socially constructed. When the two concepts of 'dying' and 'individual' are linked we are confronted with multiple interpretations of what it might mean for a person to die. 'Westernised' interpretations of individuality can vary from a death with defiance model of rebellion depicted in Dylan Thomas' poem 'Do not go gentle into that good night' (Ramsay 1975, p. 82), to the individual supremely in control of their own deathbed (Aries 1974). Foucault has added further dimensions to interpretations of the self by arguing that 'discourses', understood to be a collection of related statements or events, profoundly affect the possibilities for individual expression (Petersen 1994, p. 6). Following Foucault, we can see how discourses which promote individualism in dying may encourage the terminally ill person to make available their own subjectivity for management and control. Their grief, for example, while entirely individual, may be managed with the aid of professional support. The communal death rituals of earlier times and more traditional cultures, are consequently replaced by a privatised and professional relationship which tinges emotional subjectivity with pathology.

Individualism can be construed to be both liberating and obstructive. In the hospice–palliative care model an individual who is thought to have a Good Death interacts with others and is aware and accepting of approaching death, whereas the individual whose death is 'good enough' does it their own way but must consequently take responsibility for their own actions. Individual expression in this latter context is thought to be negative and a barrier to therapeutic intervention. This can be illustrated by the terminally ill person who refuses to discuss their approaching death and also by the dying person who may not comply with medication routines in terminal illness. Focusing on the individual, therefore, serves to provide specific treatments and support suited to the needs of each person, but it also clouds the issue of responsibility for action and inaction.

Notions of individuality also vary from culture to culture. For many Asian cultures, in particular, the individual may not be understood outside of social connectedness to others. The Confucian Chinese concept of personhood – *jen* – does not end at the boundaries of the skin but extends into the family and the intimate social circle (Kirmayer 1988, p. 78). Similarly in Japan, *ningen* – the term for person – means 'human between-ness' and defies Western individualistic notions of self (Kimura 1991, p. 235). As Kleinman (1988,

p. 11) reminds us, many members of emerging industrialised societies, as well as members of multicultural societies, may view the body as 'an open system linking social relations to the self, a vital balance between inter-related elements in a holistic cosmos'. These conceptualisations fall outside of the Cartesian mind–body split so prevalent in Western notions of the individual (Gordon 1988). It seems little wonder then, that the disjunction between Western understandings of individualism and those of many other cultural groups can complicate cross-cultural interactions in health care settings. For example, truth telling in relation to dying is not a universally held ethic. It is not unusual in a hospice and palliative care setting to find that an Italian, Greek or Chinese family will refuse to allow their dying loved one to be burdened with the knowledge about their future. Conceptualisations of self and responsibility are, in this context, vastly different from the Westernised Christian medico-centric beliefs shared by most health professionals.

Altered conceptions of self

Social construction theories of the individual or self offer explanations of how groups of people share broad understandings of what personhood means. However, these theories do not tell us a great deal about how the terminally ill person thinks and feels throughout the experience of disabling chronic illness and existential crisis. Kelly and Field (1996, pp. 250–51) suggest that bringing the body into analytical focus helps us to see the interplay between self and identity and to 'manage sociologically the relation between biological and social facts'. With this kind of conceptual framework we can see that self need not be situated 'within' the body, but 'with' the body. A significantly changed body will therefore be a significantly changed self, yet that person's sense of identity and their ability to cope with terminal illness will also continue to be linked to past experiences or 'life themes' (Zlatin 1995). The important point here is that the terminally ill person will function and think differently from the way they did when they were a healthy individual. Each person will have a unique set of circumstances which will alter their own conceptions of self and their own ability to make autonomous decisions.

Many palliative care professionals cite weakness and fatigue as one of the most disabling symptoms of terminal illness because there is little that can be done to alleviate this state of powerlessness. This manifestation of terminal illness is just one of the many symptoms which will influence the dying person's conception of themselves. Nausea, vomiting, breathlessness, constipation, diarrhoea, oedema (swelling), smell from infections and wounds, confusion and pain are also associated variously with disease and with intervention procedures. Knowledge of approaching death, whether this is implicit or explicit, and its associated anticipatory grief, further complicates self-knowledge and the capacity to act to change circumstances. It seems little wonder that the meanings of a Good Death can be vastly different for terminally ill people than for health professionals. While health professionals draw increasingly on notions of self-control and self-efficacy in their conceptualisations of 'good' and 'good enough' deaths, many terminally ill people question why dying takes so long, and as a recent study has suggested, characterise a good death as 'dying in one's sleep', 'dying quietly', 'with dignity', 'being pain free' and 'dying suddenly' (Payne et al. 1996). Nevertheless, if this is what many people want, terms like 'quietly', 'dignity' and 'suddenly' should not go unquestioned. The meanings of dignity, for example, are multiple: some people believe euthanasia is a dignified death while others believe it is unlawful killing. And what does dying 'suddenly' mean? Does the use of this word mean people would rather not have control over the circumstances of their death? Further still, the degree to which a person can be empowered or even the extent to which their wishes can be met needs to be understood in the context of social structure.

Social location and structural constraints

Any meaningful analysis of individual autonomy in decisions surrounding terminal illness and death needs to focus upon the individual's unique experience. Yet this micro-perspective needs to be understood within a structural framework which includes an understanding of each person's location within society as well as a knowledge of the macro-organisational contexts of the social world. Each individual negotiates their own illness and dying trajectories with varying degrees of ability and support due to their own place in society. The degree to which a terminally ill person has control, or is able to actively engage in decision-making has been linked to age (Rinaldi & Kearl 1990) and to patient residence and the degree to which staff set limits upon their own involvement with patients and families (Mesler 1995). Furthermore, elements which determine the terminally ill person's social location such as gender, ethnicity, social class and educational background and the kinds of social supports they receive must be understood in the light of entrenched social inequalities. The terminally ill person's access to power should also be seen in contrast to that of the health professionals who care for them. For example, a doctor who is dying of cancer can very easily negotiate their own medical management with the aid of colleagues, but an Aboriginal person is unlikely to benefit from very basic forms of support other than those provided by their own disadvantaged communities.

The inequalities of care for people suffering from terminal illnesses are institutionalised, but there is also an alarming element of chance which may affect the quality of their lives before death. We can see that a person suffering from cancer, on first consulting a doctor, begins a series of consultations, investigations and interventions, through which they will come into contact with various people who may obstruct or facilitate decisions regarding dying and death. The health professions are by no means a homogenous group. Their beliefs and actions vary greatly, particularly in this time of public and professional discussion of end of life decisions. Terminal care within Australia varies greatly: from high technology intensive care facilities to supportive hospice and palliative care services; some people die at home, but more die in nursing homes or hospitals; most people die in urban locations, while country communities suffer relative disadvantage. The degree to which a terminally ill person engages in decisions about their dying and death will therefore be mediated by their access to power and to the place and time of their death. If resources are channelled into facilities which support the needs and wishes of individuals and their families, rather than providing the latest in high technology curative treatments, people will be better able to maintain some degree of authority in the last days of their lives.

Biomedical culture, individualism and death

There have been significant changes in health professionals' responses to dying people in recent years, yet it would be premature to propose that the authority of the individual has supplanted the biomedical culture and social organisation of medicine. Medicine continues to frame the experience of individuals throughout their illness and dying trajectories. This powerful presence seems a little ironic given that medicine, with all of its technological mastery, has not wrought much change in lowering the incidence or raising the cure rates of chronic illnesses like cancer (Costain Schou 1993, p. 239). While artificial respirators and organ transplants have introduced an ambiguity about the definition and time of death, people do continue to die. However, many health professionals believe that medicine has not reached its potential for easing the burdens of dying people. Implicit in this view is the fundamental belief that if medicine cannot control death, then at the very least it should control the circumstances of death.

Even within the practice of hospice and palliative care, which proposes that death is a 'natural' part of life to be accepted when it comes, there is a very prominent view that the symptoms of dying should be treated at all cost. Some palliative care practitioners worry whether total alleviation of pain should be a goal of terminal care, yet many also are caught up with the imperative to treat and to act with whatever treatments may be current. This view may seem quite understandable when confronted with the physical devastation of diseases like terminal cancer. However, medical and cultural views of suffering overlap to obscure answers for those who seek a 'correct path' to care for dying people, particularly when that path aims to include the individual and their family in the decision-making process.

Western culture in permeated with the view that pain is growth, yet it is also very influenced by the medico-scientific approach to pain (Bendelow & Williams 1995). Most palliative care practitioners articulate a distinction between suffering and pain, but fail to conceptualise suffering in the same manner that they have contained pain within a neat neuro-physiological explanatory framework. They are far more willing than many of their colleagues in other disciplines to cross the boundary between the rationally and objectively measured sensation of pain and the lived embodied experience of pain. Yet pain that can be measured is considered a priority because this gives the impression that pain can be controlled. Additionally, measured pain serves to act as a potentially achievable audit of credibility for the health professional who must be seen to be doing their job in order to guarantee that the job will continue.

Illich (1976, p. 271) notes that in traditional cultures, '. . . pain was recognised as an inevitable part of the subjective reality of one's own body'. Such pain was made tolerable by integrating it into a meaningful setting. An original intention of the modern hospice movement, as articulated by its founder Dame Cecily Saunders (Saunders & Bains 1983, pp. 65–66), was to create an environment which was supportive to the search for meaning through pain and in the most adverse circumstances. This most fundamental philosophy is often overshadowed by the medico-scientific dimension of pain which focuses on the 'sensation' of pain rather than the meaning and experience of pain. In Australian hospice and palliative care the rhetoric of individualism must be questioned: does the control of pain by experts supersede the provision of a meaningful setting whereby the individual may learn to tolerate the sensation of pain if that is their wish? What may seem like a romanticised view here is, rather, a fundamental problem for both the terminally ill person and their professional carers. Many dying people fear pain, but also feel dissatisfied with the debilitating side effects of pain controlling medications such as morphine. The health professional may likely be faced with a dilemma: how can the terminally ill person articulate their needs and desires if their cognitive function is altered by medications, yet how can they focus on autonomous decision-making if they are incapacitated by pain? More sophisticated medications are offered as a solution, yet a cautionary note needs to be sounded about the reliance upon technology's capacity to provide answers to suffering. Overuse of medical technology will not only anaesthetise dying people to pain, it may also anaesthetise individuals to the act of dying.

The local moral world

Kleinman (1992, pp. 128–29) suggests that in order to describe and interpret interpersonal and intersubjective illness experience, ethnographers should set about conceptualising *local worlds* of illness and care. Within the local world, actions have cultural, political, economic, institutional, and social relational sources and consequences. However, local worlds need be understood as moral worlds where people recreate local patterns of *'what is most at stake* for us' in our living and dying. Following Kleinman we can see that 'what is most at stake' in the context of terminal illness may be different for individuals, yet no matter how contested or fragmented the local world is, there is a shape or coherence which makes them recognisable as a particular form of living and dying. The integrity of the terminally ill person and their capacity to assume some kind of authority over dying needs to be set within the local world. Some of the larger scale political, socioeconomic and cultural forces that impinge upon the local world of the terminally ill person have been outlined. Further moral dimensions complicate the process of deciding how dying will be managed.

The religious and cultural beliefs of the dying person, the person's family and the health professionals who care for them often influence the manner in which a terminally ill person dies. Furthermore, the philosophy and organisational culture of services for terminally ill people may constrain the degree to which the individual can make autonomous decisions. This needs to be set into a social context where the management of dying and death is highly contested. So while the Northern Territory in Australia passed legislation allowing euthanasia (July 1996), it was subsequently overturned in the Senate (March 1997). Furthermore, hospice and palliative care services have made a public stand against legalised euthanasia and presented a report which informed the Senate decision. Terminal sedation is a common practice in hospice and palliative care services, either at the request of the dying person, or at the discretion of the health professionals when the dying person is incapacitated. However, this assistance to die is not considered euthanasia as health professionals believe their intention is to alleviate the distressing symptoms of the dying person and not to deliberately end their life. If we ask the question 'what is at stake?' it becomes clear that the moral and ethical principles of a group determine the boundaries of individual authority over dying.

Conclusion

The preceding discussion has illustrated many of the concerns that face dying people, their families and their health professional carers. While the micro-context of each terminally ill person's experience of suffering and their ability to be involved in decision-making at the end of life is unique, it must also be situated within historical, social and cultural contexts. These contexts inform our understanding of what it means to die, as well as influencing the degree to which we may be able to participate in the circumstances of our deaths. Individual characteristics cannot fully explain the circumstances of each person's experience of dying. So rather than proposing that the terminally ill person might have a 'good' or 'good enough' death based upon their capacity for interpersonal interaction and autonomous decision-making, an alternative way of looking at the dying and death may be to consider it 'good enough' relative to social as well as individual factors.

Many of the factors that influence the individual's experience of dying are social: the social location of the individual and their access to power; cultural understandings of dying, death and individuality; the political and economic organisation of medicine and health care; and the moral dimensions of shared decision-making. Yet the actual experience of terminal illness is also embodied and personal. A person who experiences terminal illness and approaching death will be changed by the experience. The experience is not a series of isolated events, but a process of deterioration, interrupted by unpredictable changes and re-evaluations. If each person's death is considered as unique relative to the kinds of considerations that have been outlined in this chapter we will be better able to acknowledge individual agency, structural constraint, culture and change.

While a growing body of literature in the sociology of dying, death and bereavement has contributed to our understanding of death in advanced industrialised society, further socially-oriented research is needed to elaborate the social and the embodied experience of dying. This is particularly important in view of the fact that most deaths in advanced industrial societies occur as the result of long-term disease conditions where it is likely that people will be aware of their approaching death. This chapter goes some way towards conceptualising issues that are of concern to all those who value individual empowerment in end of life decision-making.

Note

1 The terminology used to describe the kinds of societies Australians, New Zealanders, British and North Americans live in is often disputed in social science discourse. The term 'Western' is thought to convey a geographical meaning which is inappropriate in the context of changing and globalising forces. Yet a term is needed to describe the influence of certain kinds of philosophical thought that have contributed to contemporary knowledge. In this latter case I have used the term 'Western'. Elsewhere I have employed the terms 'advanced' and 'emerging' industrialised countries, both of which may be multicultural to varying degrees.

References

Aries, P. 1974 *Western Attitudes to Death,* Johns Hopkins University Press, Baltimore, MA.
—— 1981 *The Hour of Our Death,* Allen Lane, London.
Bauman, Z. 1992 *Mortality, Immortality and Other Life Strategies,* Polity Press, Cambridge.
Baume, P. 1993 'Living and dying: A paradox in medical progress', *The Medical Journal of Australia* vol. 159, pp. 792–94.
Bendelow, G. & Williams, S. 1995 'Transcending the dualisms: Towards a sociology of pain', *Sociology of Health and Illness* vol. 17, no. 2, pp. 139–65.
Campbell, A. 1990 'An ethic for hospice', paper presented at The Australian Hospice and Palliative Care Conference, Adelaide, 22 November.
Cassell, E. 1975 'Dying in a technological society', in *Death Inside Out: The Hastings Centre Report,* eds P. Steinfels & R. Veatch, Harper & Row, New York.
Costain Schou, K. 1993 'Awareness contexts and the construction of dying in the cancer treatment setting: "Micro" and "macro" levels in narrative analysis', in *The Sociology of Death: Theory, Culture, Practice,* ed. D. Clark, Blackwell, Oxford.
Elias, N. 1985 *The Loneliness of Dying,* Blackwell, Oxford.
Gavin, W. 1995 *Cuttin' the Body Loose: Historical, Biological, and Personal Approaches to Death and Dying,* Temple University Press, Philadelphia.

Gordon, D. 1988 'Tenacious assumptions in Western medicine', in *Biomedicine Examined*, eds M. Lock & D. Gordon, Kluwer Academic Publishers, Dordrecht.

Gorer, G. 1965 *Death, Grief and Mourning in Contemporary Britain*, Cresset, London.

Hunt, R. 1994 'Palliative care – the rhetoric–reality gap' in *Willing to Listen Wanting to Die*, ed. H. Kuhse, Penguin Books, Ringwood.

Illich, I. 1976 *Limits to Medicine. Medical Nemesis: The Expropriation of Health*, Marion Boyars, London.

Kellehear, A. 1984 'Are we a "death-denying" society? A sociological review', *Social Science and Medicine* vol. 18, no. 9, pp. 713–23.

—— 1996 *Experiences Near Death: Beyond Medicine and Religion*, Oxford University Press, Oxford.

Kelner, M. & Bourgeault, I. 1993 'Patient control over dying: Responses of health care professionals', *Social Science and Medicine* vol. 36, no. 6, pp. 757–65.

Kelly, M. & Field, D. 1996 'Medical sociology, chronic illness and the body', *Sociology of Health and Illness* vol. 18, no. 2, pp. 241–57.

Kimura, R. 1991 'Fiduciary relationships and the medical profession: A Japanese point of view', in *Ethics, Trust, and the Professions: Philosophical and Cultural Aspects*, eds E. Pellegrino, R. Veatch & J. Langan, Georgetown University Press, Washington.

Kirmayer, L. 1988 'Mind and body as metaphors: Hidden values in biomedicine', in *Biomedicine Examined*, eds M. Lock & D. Gordon, Kluwer Academic Publishers, Netherlands.

Kleinman, A. 1988 *The Illness Narratives: Suffering, Healing and the Human Condition*, Basic Books, New York.

—— 1992 'Local worlds of suffering: An interpersonal focus for ethnographies of illness experience', *Qualitative Health Research* vol. 2, no. 2, pp. 127–34.

Komesaroff, P., Norelle Lickiss, J., Parker, M. & Ashby, M. 1995 'The euthanasia controversy: Decision making in extreme cases', *The Medical Journal of Australia* vol. 162, pp. 594–97.

Lock, M. 1996 'Death in technological time: Locating the end of meaningful life', *Medical Anthropology Quarterly* vol. 10, no. 4, pp. 575–600.

McNamara, B., Waddell, C. & Colvin, M. 1994 'The institutionalisation of the Good Death', *Social Science and Medicine* vol. 39, no. 11, pp. 1501–8.

—— 1995 'Threats to the Good Death: The cultural context of stress and coping among hospice nurses', *Sociology of Health and Illness* vol. 17, no. 2, pp. 222–44.

Mellor, P. 1993 'Death in high modernity: The contemporary presence and absence of death', in *The Sociology of Death: Theory, Culture, Practice*, ed. D. Clark, Blackwell, Oxford.

Mellor, P. & Shilling, C. 1993 'Modernity, self-identity and the sequestration of death', *Sociology* vol. 27, no. 3, pp. 411–31.

Mesler, M. 1995 'The philosophy and practice of patient control in hospice: The dynamics of autonomy versus paternalism', *Omega* vol. 30, no. 3, pp. 173–89.

Metcalf, P. & Huntington, R. 1991 *Celebrations of Death: The Anthropology of Mortuary Ritual*, 2nd edn, Cambridge University Press, Cambridge.

Moller, D. 1990 *On Death Without Dignity: The Human Impact of Technological Dying*, Baywood Publishing, New York.

Muller, J. & Koenig, B. 1988 'On the boundary of life and death: The definition of dying by medical residents', in *Biomedicine Examined*, eds M. Lock & D. Gordon, Kluwer Academic Publishers, Netherlands.

Nuland, S. 1994 *How We Die: Reflections on Life's Final Chapter,* Chatto & Windus, London.

Parsons, T., Fox, R. & Lidz, V. 1972 'The "gift of life" and its reciprocation', *Social Research* vol. 39, pp. 367–415.

Payne, S., Langley-Evans, A. & Hillier, R. 1996 'Perceptions of a "good" death: A comparative study of the views of hospice staff and patients', *Palliative Medicine* vol. 10, pp. 307–12.

Petersen, A. 1994 *In A Critical Condition: Health and Power Relations in Australia,* Allen & Unwin, Sydney.

Ramsay, P. 1975 'The indignity of death with dignity', in *Death Inside Out: The Hastings Centre Report,* eds P. Steinfels & R. Veatch, Harper & Row, New York.

Rinaldi, A. & Kearl, M. 1990 'The hospice farewell: Ideological perspectives of its professional practitioners', *Omega* vol. 21, no. 4, pp. 283–300.

Saunders, C. & Baines, M. 1983 *Living With Dying: The Management of Terminal Disease,* Oxford University Press, Oxford.

Veatch, R. 1976 *Death, Dying and the Biological Revolution,* Yale University Press, Connecticut.

Waddell, C., Clarnette, R., Smith, M., Oldham, L. & Kellehear, A. 1996 'Treatment decision-making at the end of life: A survey of Australian doctors' attitudes towards patients' wishes and euthanasia', *The Medical Journal of Australia* vol. 165, pp. 540–44.

Walters, T. 1991 'Modern death: Taboo or not taboo?', *Sociology* vol. 25, no. 2, pp. 293–310.

Zlatin, D. 1995 'Life themes: A method to understand terminal illness', *Omega* vol. 31, no. 3, pp. 189–206.

Index

Sontag, S. 228
Southwood Smith, Dr. 10–11
spectacles 15–16
Sri Lankan health policy 54
Starr, P. 140, 142
starvation 159, 160
state: bureaucracies 4; family policy 36,
    37–8; health improvements 50;
    poverty 86, 91; power 137; private
    live 36; professions 135, 136–7,
    138–9, 140–1; *see also* welfare benefits
state intervention 37, 126, 136–7
stigma: courtesy stigma 181, 208–9,
    214–15; disease 133; families
    208–15; management 210–14;
    neutralisation 211, 213
Stimson, G. 180
Stott, N. C. H. 185, 186
Strauss, A. 206
stress management: cigarette smoking
    181–2, 223–5; *see also* psychological
    stress
strokes 47, 90
Strong, P. M. 204
structure/agency 63, 103–6
sulphonamides 159–60, 162
The Sun 231, 233
sunbathing 230
Supporting Families (Home Office) 5,
    36–40
Sure Start (DfEE) 5
surveillance medicine 127, 144, 148,
    149–50; *see also* self-surveillance
Susman, W. 233
Sydney Morning Herald 152
symbolic goods 105
symbolism, diagnostic testing 156–7
syphilis 90
Szasz, Thomas S. 131

Tancredi, L. 151, 153
taxation: family income 37; National
    Health Service 27, 31; welfare state
    67
technological development: death 247,
    253; individualism 246
telephones 219–20
terminally ill people: Australia 244–5,
    251–2; autonomy 248; body 254–5;

empowerment 247, 255; local moral
    world 253–4; self 250–1; social
    location 251–2
Thatcher, Margaret 4, 5, 140, 141
third way: communitarianism 5–7;
    health improvements 49; National
    Health Service 41–6; universalism 6
Thomas, Dylan 249
Thomas, H. E. 74
toilet training 238–40
town planning 140–1
Townsend, P. 61–2, 64
tribalism in medical profession 128,
    164, 170–1
truancy 38
tuberculosis 92, 146, 150, 161
Tudor Hart, J. 61
Turner, B. 238, 239, 241, 242
Turner, B. S. 231
Turner, Lana 231
typhus 10, 12

UAW 100
UK Royal College of Practitioners
    90
Ulanowsky, C. 156
ultrasound scanning 154
unemployment 78–80, 86, 113
UNICEF 92
United Nations 88, 89, 92
universalism: classical 6, 53; National
    Health Service 61; new 6, 56–7;
    third way 6
universities: competition 174–5; market
    forces 174; publications 174–5;
    research 173–6
urbanisation 3, 8–9, 161, 163
US: health insurance 54; health
    screening 147–8; health services 32,
    96, 153, 167; life expectancy of
    women 88–9; longevity/gender 90;
    poverty/health 95–6; race/health
    90; social class 107; victim blaming
    62; women's health 89; *see also*
    Anglo-Saxon people; Irish people;
    Italian people
US National Institutes of Health 88, 89,
    90
user groups, health services 128–9